Building A Better World Together
A Career in Women's Health

Linda Andrews, BSN, MPH
Nurse Practitioner in Women's Health

Cover Art: Susanne Peck

Proceeds from the sale of this book will go to the Jean Andrews Nursing Scholarship Fund; funds are raised by the Porter Hospital Auxiliary, Middlebury, Vermont, and administered by the Vermont Student Assistance Corporation.

Bristol Press LLC
Bristol, VT 05443

ISBN: 979-8-3881478-8-2

I dedicate this book to my Grandparents; Isabelle "Belle" Stewart Andrews, Dr. Ralph Randall Stewart, and my parents Jean Stewart Andrews and Dr. Bertrand Joel Andrews. They were my inspiration and support that enabled me to have a career in international health. I am eternally grateful.

Linda Andrews

Notable Quotes

"It's exciting and refreshing to see such a wonderful piece written by a University of Vermont nursing alumnus – any healthcare provider or student who reads this will be revitalized by seeing what one woman has accomplished through her international experiences!"

Rosemary Dale
University of Vermont Chair of Nursing
Associate Dean for Clinical Practice

"If I had read this book when I was younger, it would have changed my life."

Diane Cushman
Retired Public Health Nurse
Graduate of Vanderbilt University

Preface

I am writing my memoirs for those interested in pursuing an international health career. This book describes my life experiences of nearly thirty years working in Africa and Asia; long term in seven different countries and short term in five others. I share how I became interested in an international career and my "road map" on how I qualified to work in international health, found my positions, settled into new countries, my work experiences, and how I entertained myself. I am also writing this for my family and friends so they can better understand what I was doing for all those years away from home.

This book describes a point in time in each country. I describe what I view as key or interesting accomplishments with a focus on my collaborative style and my role as an expatriate. I do not go into the political history of each country, but may briefly discuss some sensitive issues that had an impact on me.

I used full names and pictures of people only when I received permission. If I was unable to get permission, I used first names, substitute names, initials, or just their position title. I also used a picture if it was taken in a public setting.

Linda Andrews

Table of Contents

Forward

Linda and I grew up together in Middlebury, Vermont. We went to kindergarten, elementary, and high school together. We went to different colleges, but had similar career paths and have remained close friends throughout our lives. I went to the College of Wooster in Ohio where I majored in history and Linda went to the University of Vermont to study nursing. After college, we were both in each other's weddings; I was married first and when Linda married, she wore my wedding dress!

We spent our careers loving to travel and working in developing countries. I was an educator and eventually dean at Northfield Mount Hermon, a private high school in Massachusetts, for forty-one years. I had the satisfaction of developing the school's international programs and was able to travel and learn with students. My family has a camp for girls, Betsey Cox, and for boys, Camp Sangamon, in Pittsford, Vermont, and I now own and co-direct Camp Betsey Cox. One of my objectives is to have campers get to know and understand people from other countries and cultures. I hire counselors and staff from around the world, offering the campers an international experience.

For nearly thirty years, Linda worked in twelve countries, seven long-term assignments and five as a short-term consultant for various international organizations. I visited her when she was working in Bangladesh with the United States Agency for International Development. We traveled together in Nepal, hiking in the foothills of Mt. Everest, and riding elephants to see rare rhinos. I later studied Islam on a sabbatical, traveling to many Islamic countries, and Linda worked in many Islamic countries, too, another area from which we have developed a mutual respect for the people of the Islamic faith.

When Linda turned seventy, she was diagnosed with stage 4B uterine cancer with a 17 percent chance of living past five years. She had a counselor at the UVM Medical Center, Dr. Shira Louria, who helped navigate through her fears of cancer and listened to Linda talk about her love and passion of her international work. Dr. Louria, as well as myself and many of her friends, encouraged her to write down her adventures and I offered to help. I sat with her during her many chemotherapy treatments and recorded her stories. Good news! Linda has now been cancer-free since 2017! We decided to finalize these stories for those interested in an international health career or who have an interest in hearing the lessons she learned after all her years of working in Asia and Africa.

In editing her work and finding photos for this book, we have shared a lot and have become even closer friends.

Lorrie Byrom

Abbreviations

AIDS	Acquired Immune Deficiency Syndrome
AMW	Auxiliary Midwife
ARV	Antiretroviral
AVSC	Association for Voluntary Surgical Contraception
CARs	Central Asian Republics
DHS	Demographic Health Survey
DYC	Dar es Salaam Yacht Club
EGPAF	Elizabeth Glaser Pediatric AIDs Foundation
FH	Family Health
FHD	Family Health Division
FP	Family Planning
FPCST	Family Planning Clinical Supervisory Team
FWV	Family Welfare Visitor
FSG	Family Support Group
ICAP	International Center for AIDS Care and Treatment Program
IUD	Intrauterine Device
JSI	John Snow, Inc
MCH	Maternal and Child Health
MOH	Ministry of Health
NGO	Non-Governmental Organization
NIPORT	National Institute for Population Research and Training
HIV	Human Immunodeficiency Virus
HPV	Human Papilloma Virus
PEPFAR	President's Emergency Plan of AIDS Relief
PMTCT	Prevention of Mother to Child Transmission
PSC	Personal Service Contractor
PSG	Peer Support Group
SEVIA	Smartphone Enhanced Visual Inspection with Acetic Acid
STI	Sexually Transmitted Infection

SWDO	Somali Women's Democratic Organization
TSE	Training, Supervision and Education Section
USAID	United States Agency for International Development
VIA	Visual Inspection with Acetic Acid
WHO	World Health Organization

Introduction

"Life Isn't About Finding Yourself,
Life is About Creating Yourself."

George Bernard Shaw

Creating Myself: Genetics or Environment?

I grew up in the small town of Middlebury, Vermont. On my paternal side, I come from three generations of medical doctors in Vermont. My father, Dr. Bertrand Joel (B.J), Andrews, worked as a family physician at our local hospital, Porter Hospital, for thirty-five years. He delivered more than 5,000 babies in our county! My grandfather, Dr. Bertrand Fletcher (B.F.) Andrews, made many house calls and in the winter would go by horse and sleigh to visit his patients! My great-grandfather, Dr. Bertrand Joel Andrews, was the fifth medical superintendent of the Mary Fletcher Hospital in Burlington, Vermont.

My mother, Jean Stewart Andrews, was born in Sialkot, India, on March 9, 1919. She was home-schooled in Rawalpindi, and went to high school at Woodstock, an international boarding school located in the foothills of the Himalayas. She graduated from University of Vermont (UVM) majoring in psychology. She worked at the Brandon Training School, a school for people with developmental disabilities and it was where she met my father, who was working as a UVM medical intern. They married and raised three children: Joel, Jim, and myself. Mom was very active volunteering in the community. She worked with the Porter Hospital Auxiliary, where she helped to establish the Grey Ladies and the Junior Nursing Aides. I was

5

trained as a Junior Nursing Aide and had my first experience working in a hospital. Before she died on April 13, 1970, the Auxiliary honored her by establishing the Jean Andrews Nursing Scholarship (JANS) fund. According to her obituary, "she was deeply interested in the nursing profession and aware of the need for registered nurses and licensed practical nurses to be trained." More than fifty years later, this fund is still active, providing scholarships every year to residents of Addison County! I recently became a donor to this fund--better late than never!

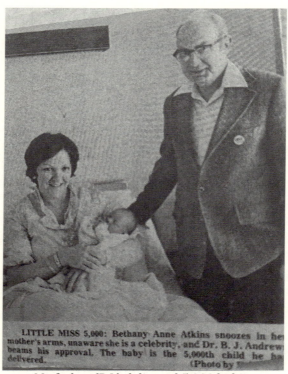

LITTLE MISS 5,000: Bethany Anne Atkins snoozes in her mother's arms, unaware she is a celebrity, and Dr. B. J. Andrews beams his approval. The baby is the 5,000th child he has delivered.
(Photo by ...)

My father (B.J.) delivered 5,000 babies
in Addison County, Vermont.

My maternal grandparents were both raised in upstate New York. My grandmother, Isabelle (Belle) Caroline Darrow, met my grandfather, Ralph Randall Stewart, when going to graduate school at Columbia University. Both had just finished three-year stints teaching in United Presbyterian Missionary Colleges abroad. My grandmother was getting her Master in Arts and my grandfather his Ph.D. in Botany. After they graduated, they married in Middlebury in 1916 and moved to Rawalpindi, India (now Pakistan) to work at a well-known and respected United Presbyterian missionary college called Gordon College. My grandfather was a professor of Botany and eventually became the college president. My grandmother became Dean of Women. They lived in Rawalpindi for forty-three years from 1917 to 1960.

My grandfather, Dr R. R. Stewart. is famous for doing the baseline survey of the plants in the Himalayas. He and my grandmother spent summers traveling by horseback in the Himalayas collecting plants. When he retired, he gave his collection of 50,000 plants specimens to Gordon College. The "Stewart Collection" is now in Pakistan's National Herbarium at Islamabad. He is well known for his work, which is documented at Kew Gardens in London. He eventually retired in Duarte, California, to a retirement home for Presbyterian missionaries. When he was 100 years old, he was invited to fly to Rawalpindi to give the opening and closing speeches at an international botanical conference. His speech focused on the impact of population growth on the environment. My aunt and my two brothers flew in from the States and I flew in from Somalia to see him honored and to hear his speeches. Grandfather lived until he was 103.

My grandmother, Isabelle Darrow, known as Belle, was a strong and independent woman who spent her life teaching internationally. She strongly believed in female education.

When she was Dean of Women at Gordon College, she was recorded as saying "that she was fighting a battle against women's slavery and ignorance." Belle graduated from Middlebury College in 1911, and before she met my grandfather, she had traveled to Marsovan, Turkey, for a three-year position teaching science at Anatolia College, which was run by the United Presbyterian Church. It had primarily Turkish and Armenian Christian students and faculty. In 1914, the Armenian Genocide took place; Islamic Turkish nationalists used the cover of the First World War to wipe out the Christian Armenian population. Around 1.5 million Armenians were massacred. We are not sure where Belle was at this time, but she ended up in Constantinople (now Istanbul) and worked at a Turkish hospital until the United States Ambassador to the Ottoman Empire arranged for her and a few other Americans to return to the United States through Bulgaria. She learned that many of her Armenian students, teachers, and friends from Anatolia College were murdered. Grandfather said she never talked about the tragedy she witnessed in Turkey. [1] She died at the age of 63 in 1953. She is buried in Rawalpindi and I visited the gravesite when I went to hear grandfather speak at the conference.

With three generations of physicians on my paternal side and two generations on my maternal side having lived and/or worked in developing countries, I think genetics may have played a major role in my desire to work in international health.

---

[1] Information on Jean Andrews, Elizabeth Darrow, and Dr. R. R. Stewart came from *This Family*, written by William Darrow.

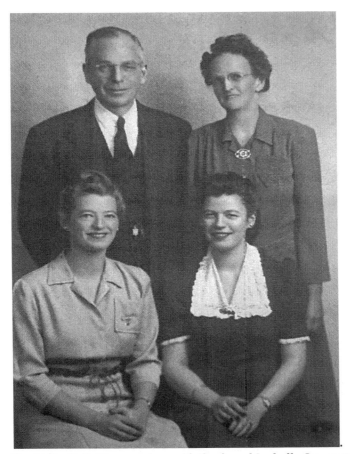

Back: Dr. R. R. Stewart (grandfather) and Isabelle Stewart (grandmother) / Front: Jean Andrews (mother) and Ellen Daniels (aunt).

Creating Myself Through Education and Experience to Work Internationally

It was in second grade, while walking in a Halloween parade dressed as a nurse, that I made the decision to become a missionary nurse in India. When making life choices while growing up, I always asked myself, will this training and

9

experience make me qualified to work internationally? While I didn't become a missionary, I did become a nurse and worked internationally in more than twelve countries with different governmental and non-governmental organizations.

I got my nursing degree from the University of Vermont (UVM) in 1969. In my junior year, one of my nursing instructors encouraged me to apply to the Frontier Nursing Service, located in the Appalachian Mountains of Kentucky. I applied and spent the summer of my junior year working in this very rural setting with extreme poverty. Appalachia had a unique culture with its own music and dance, which I loved, and a dialect that was difficult to understand. I worked first in a rural hospital which was an old converted house and later in an outpost working with a nurse midwife. The midwives use to make house visits by horseback, but now Jeeps were used. I learned to drive a Jeep, dry my brakes after traversing rivers, and find my way up "hollers" to visit patients in tar-paper shacks. I had to avoid feuding families and turn a blind eye to the stills making moonshine. This gave me my first "third world experience" and cemented my desire to work in developing countries.

After I graduated from UVM, I gained experience as a staff nurse at Boston University Hospital, Washington University Hospital in Seattle, and then worked in a small rural hospital in Anacortes, Washington. I attained skills in public health by working as a public health and school nurse in the San Juan Islands off the coast of Washington State.

I received a Women's Health Care Nurse Practitioner certificate in 1974. While working in the San Juan Islands, I was offered free training as a women's health care nurse practitioner if I agreed to work at a Planned Parenthood in Bellingham, Washington, for two years. I loved this work and went on to be an instructor to train women's health care nurse practitioners in Seattle. Here I gained experience in teaching adult nursing students, providing both didactic and clinical training. With these skills, I was asked to be a consultant for the State of Washington to develop quality care standards for family planning clinics. This was a great job where I learned to work with state governments, setting standards, assessing clinics, and providing technical assistance when needed.

I had learned that most international agencies working in health required a Master's in Public Health (MPH). I was now thirty-five years old! I had been married and divorced, had ended a long-term partnership, and decided the time was right to get my degree and to start my international career! But I was very nervous about giving up a great job with all the benefits. Encouraged by a former UVM instructor, I left my job and in 1984 got my MPH in International Health at the University of California, Los Angeles (UCLA). One of my proudest moments was when my grandfather, Dr. R. R. Stewart, attended my graduation where I received two awards: The Dean L. S. Goerke Memorial Award for Recognition of Outstanding Achievement in Graduate Studies in Public Health, and the School of Public Health Alumni Association Award for outstanding academic achievement, character, leadership, extra-curricular involvement, and service to the University of California, Los Angeles.

I now had the academic credentials but I had another hurdle to overcome. While at UCLA, I learned that most international agencies required two years living overseas. Most of the students in my master's program had two years in the Peace Corps. I had no international experience. So as part of my master's program, I secured funding to spend three months in Tamil Nadu, India, teaching IUD insertions for midwives in a rural primary health care center. This center was associated with the Christian Medical College in Vellore where they trained physicians and nurses in primary care. I loved every minute of it!

After I graduated with my MPH, I was able to get a short-term consultancy working in Nigeria introducing family planning into the nursing schools in Imo State. This involved training the nurse midwife tutors and developing a curriculum and training materials. I traveled and worked with an experienced consultant who taught me important lessons on how to train cross culturally. However, I still needed a long-term assignment. After much searching, I was fortunate to find and be offered a two-year population service internship with the University of Michigan working in Thailand with the Family Health Division (FHD) of the Ministry of Health! After my internship, the FHD asked me to extend my stay for another nine months.

Following my internship, I had no trouble finding international work. I applied for each new job and worked as a contractor for a variety of organizations. I worked long term in Thailand, Somalia, Bangladesh, Central Asia Republics, Malawi, Uganda, and Tanzania, and had short-term assignments in Rwanda, Mozambique, and Ghana. Looking back, it was helpful to start international work in my forties after I had completed my formal education, had gained many valuable experiences and had developed skills that I could share.

Linda Andrews's Long-Term Assignments

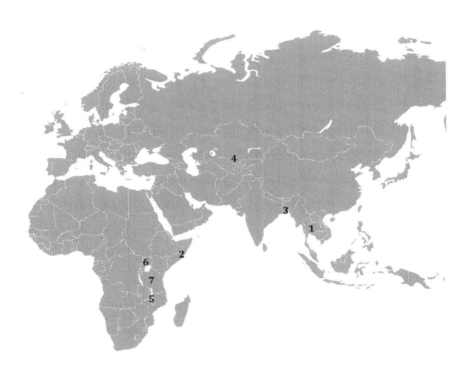

1 Thailand
2 Somalia
3 Bangladesh
4 Central Asia Republics
5 Malawi
6 Uganda
7 Tanzania

Thailand
September 1985-June 1988

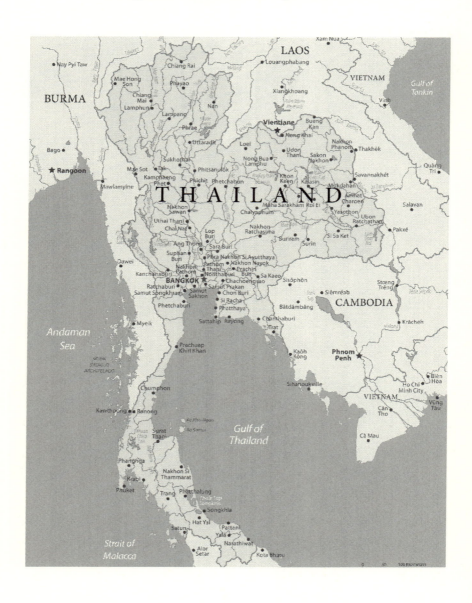

My First International Position

My first international posting was as a Population Service Intern offered by the School of Public Health, University of Michigan. It was a USAID (United States Agency for International Development) supported program, designed to provide overseas experience to prepare graduates for careers in international health. It was the perfect program for me! I was now thirty-eight years old, a nurse practitioner in women's health care with my master's degree in public health; this program was a great opportunity for me to get long term international experience. I applied and was offered a two-year internship in Thailand! I would be working in the Training, Supervision, and Education Section (TSE) of the Family Health Division (FHD), Department of Health in the Ministry of Health (MOH).

Settling In: Overcoming Culture Shock

In September of 1985, I traveled to Bangkok. I was very anxious about living overseas for two years. I was met at the airport by my Thai supervisors from the Training, Supervision and Education Section. They drove me to a hotel where I stayed until they found a lovely furnished three-bedroom townhouse for me in a quiet, wealthy neighborhood. It was owned by King Rama's great granddaughter, a princess of the royal family!

When I arrived, I didn't know anyone, didn't speak Thai, did not know how to use their public transportation, had never eaten Thai food, and I knew very little about the culture. I felt very disconnected from my friends and family in the United States. I had a landline, but telephone calls were very expensive; there were no cell phones or computers, thus no emails. My communication with home was mainly by handwritten letters. I felt lonely, disoriented, and uneasy.

I was experiencing culture shock. A professor from Evergreen College, who was visiting Thailand, paid me a visit, and explained that when you move into a different culture, you lose definition of yourself; your friends, language, food, housing, transport, pets, etc. are what define you as a person. When you change all that at once, you go through culture shock.

Unknowingly, I found ways to overcome this. When I moved into my townhouse, I asked two young Thai women to come live with me for a few months to help me with shopping, cooking, and getting around the city. I later hired a Thai woman, Nit, to cook and clean for me. Nit ended up being great company and stayed with me for three years. She only cooked Thai cuisine, so after adjusting to spicy foods, I learned to love her cooking. She introduced me to strange looking fruits like rambutan, jackfruit, and mangosteen, which were delicious. I even acquired the taste for one of the most popular Thai fruits called durian, a fruit that smells like dirty socks. To make the townhouse feel more like my home, Nit took me to the public market where I bought some pets. I bought a rose-ringed parakeet, who was quite smart and entertaining, but eventually flew away. I bought a fish tank and filled it with tropical fish and two white rabbits that reminded me of my Angora rabbits I raised at home.

Making friends was my key to settling in and I made some very good ones at work. Two of them had their master's degrees in public health and were fluent in English. We called ourselves The Three Musketeers: Tassanee, Dang, and I. Tassanee was an excellent tennis player and insisted I learn to play. She connected me with an instructor who spoke only Thai, so this was the beginning of my language training! She also took me to

16

her beauty salon, where I had my first face massage, pedicure, and manicure! She introduced me to inexpensive but delicious street food and taught me how to judge what was safe to eat. Besides my friends at work, I made friends by attending an international Christian church and joined a choir that sang Handel's "Messiah" at Christmas with a full orchestra! I also met and became very close friends with some of the Peace Corps staff. During the holidays, we had a great time traveling together to Burma and later to Hong Kong.

In the beginning, getting around Bangkok was a challenge since I didn't have a car. Tassanee drove me around, but I knew I would have to start using public transportation. Few people spoke English so I had to learn how to give directions and negotiate a price in Thai. I was able to learn how to travel by water taxi, bus, or tuk tuk, a three-wheeled motorized vehicle. In those days, there was little traffic and it was easy to get around.

I struggled with learning the Thai language, so I enrolled in language training at the American University Alumni School. I found it a very difficult language to grasp, but I learned the basics: polite greetings, how to negotiate the cost of items, order food, give directions, etc. Since speaking the language was difficult for me, my Thai colleagues practiced their English with me. One of my colleagues, who had limited English language skills when I met her, became so proficient she applied and got into a Master's in Public Health program in the United States!

Looking back, I realize I had very little knowledge of the Thai culture and learned how important it was to understand the culture in order to build relationships and work effectively. I would say the most important thing I learned was to smile. Thailand is sometimes called "The Land of the Smiles." Thais are welcoming and friendly and try to avoid confrontation and the expression of negative emotions. I learned that Thais will not say "no." I would get a nod of agreement and maybe even a "yes" on some proposed action and then be surprised when nothing happened. I would later learn that there was a good reason for not following up on an action. There were many non-verbal gestures that were important to learn, like never touch someone's head or point your feet at anyone. When sitting in a Buddhist temple, I had to carefully sit with my feet pointing away from the Buddha. A respectful gesture was to hand an object or paper to someone by holding it out in your right hand while placing your left hand under your right elbow. I also learned to bow with hands together when greeting older people and those in senior positions.

The Thai work ethic also was different than what I was accustomed. The women in the office dressed smartly with Western-style dresses and shoes with heels. I felt very underdressed. My Thai friends took me to a tailor where I had suits designed and custom made to fit me. I also had to adjust to not having my weekends free; Thai work days and weekends were not clearly defined. Work was integrated with play. When we traveled for work, there always was time to visit the monasteries and temples and to give respect to the prominent monks.

Singing was a big part of the culture. Many times, after a day of work, we would have dinner together and sing. Everyone was expected to sing a solo on stage including me! I dreaded this, because I could never think of a song not to mention remember the words, so I came prepared with a song and carried the words with me. My biggest hit was singing "Proud Mary!"

Sometimes when traveling, they would take me to these very popular cabaret shows performed by Katoeys, transgender women or effeminate gay men. The shows took place on a stage with great music, fabulous singing, and dancing. The performers wore outrageous costumes with extreme makeup.

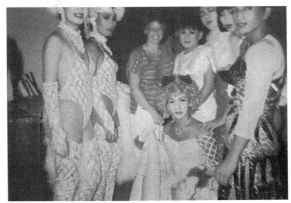

Linda with Katoey dancers.

The Thai staff also planned and enjoyed staff retreats. I was invited to a very special retreat that included an overnight ferry ride to a remote island for swimming and snorkeling. I was stunned by the pristine beauty of the coral reefs and fish.

I studied Buddhism since Theravada Buddhism was followed by 95 percent of the population. I took classes, visited many monasteries, and observed Buddhist practices. I spent a few weekends at a wat, a place of worship, meditating with my American friend who was becoming a Buddhist nun. She had shaven her head, wore the traditional white robe of the nuns, and had been practicing meditation for the last seven years. I enjoyed this time with her, but was disturbed to see the way the nuns were subservient to the male monks, such as preparing the monk's food and eating after they ate.

My Thai friends celebrated their birthdays by offering the monks food in the morning as they walked by holding bowls in which to accept offerings. Then during the day, they would go to a wat and give an offering to the resident monk(s). When I turned forty, I told Dang I wanted to give an offering to a Buddhist nun not the monks. We then went to visit one of the oldest wats in Bangkok. There were fifty to one hundred monks chanting in front of an old Buddha statue with one older nun sitting there. I first lit a candle and incense and then put a small gold-leaf flake on the Buddha. Dang then explained to the nun that it was my birthday and I wanted to offer her money. She accepted and offered me a prayer. I was emotionally moved; with the monks chanting, the candle lit, the incense going, and the nun offering me a prayer, it was a very special fortieth birthday. One of my supervisors called me a Protestant-Buddhist.

Work Experience

I later realized how fortunate I was to have been offered this internship. I had the invaluable experience of working at the national level within the Ministry of Health. It was a unique position, because the Family Health Division (FHD) of the Ministry of Health, requested and approved my application! My education, experience, and skills were wanted!

I accepted this position thinking I would be working in the family planning program. However, during my orientation, I learned they already had an established and quality family planning program and they wanted me to improve their well-child clinics. I am embarrassed to say I resisted; I argued that I was a nurse practitioner in women's health, not well-child care.

In the Thai style to avoid any confrontation, I was invited on a field trip so I could see these clinics first-hand. I was surprised to see women with their babies lined up outdoors. The babies were weighed on scales hanging from a tree, the weight was recorded on a growth chart, and then given immunizations. There was no health education for the mother and no physical examination or advice on the child's physical and mental development.

I later learned that before I had arrived in Thailand, the government had declared 1986 to be the year to promote maternal and child health. As a result of this policy, the Department of Health formed a special committee to improve maternal and child health services. They conducted a survey that found more than a quarter of children under five suffered from malnutrition, one of the main causes responsible for infant mortality. They knew and reported that the well-child care services, which was provided by the auxiliary midwives in the health centers, were substandard.

The Family Health Division determined the best way to remedy this situation was to train the auxiliary midwives (AMWs) in well-child care, which would include the child's physical, mental, and social development. The AMWs would be trained to train village health workers, traditional birth attendants, and "model" mothers to give advice on well-child care and when to refer children for health services. Finally, nurse district supervisors would be trained to ensure the provision of quality care by these different cadres of health providers.

Now that I understood the need and what needed to be done, what could I do? I didn't have any expertise in well-child care. I then found the obvious solution; I would ask the experts: the Thai pediatricians. With support from my supervisors, I wrote a proposal to the World Health Organization (WHO), requesting funding to organize a conference with key pediatricians and government officials. I was so excited when WHO agreed to fund this conference!

As a result of the conference, a medical advisory committee was formed which set standards for the well-child care services. It defined the roles of the district nurse supervisors, auxiliary midwives, and the other cadres of health care providers in the village. The committee developed curricula, determined the necessary supplies and equipment needed in the health centers, developed health care records and a health card for the mother.

The next step was to design a program and write a proposal for funding the implementation and evaluation of a well-child care project. I learned there were six maternal and child centers that provided update/refresher training for the auxiliary midwives working in the health centers. It was decided to pilot this program at those centers.

As we were designing the program, I met a former Peace Corps volunteer who was now employed in the research division of the Ministry of Health. He advised me to write the proposal as an operational research project. We determined we needed thirty-six experimental health centers and nine control health centers to measure the success of the well-child care program. With his knowledge and expertise, we developed tools for a baseline assessment and a survey that included a chart audit and interviews with mothers. An evaluation task force would conduct a three-, six-, and twelve-month evaluation.

One of my biggest challenges was developing a budget for the proposal. I had no idea of the cost of training, supplies, and equipment. Thankfully, my immediate supervisor helped me work out a budget.

With consultation from my supervisors, I wrote a two-year proposal for this pilot project called "Improvement of Well-Child Clinic Services Project." The next challenge was to find an organization to fund it. I went with my supervisors to various organizations where we presented the proposal and requested funding. We were thrilled when Redd Barna, Norwegian Save the Children, agreed to provide funding. My role was to facilitate the implementation and assist in the evaluation of this pilot program.

Throughout the next two years, I enjoyed traveling with my colleagues to all the Maternal and Child Health (MCH) centers, observing the trainings and visiting the health centers. At the completion of the project, all six MCH centers had qualified instructors and trained district nurses as supervisors in well-child care. The AMWs in the 36 experimental health centers had been trained in a ten-day course. The AMWs had returned to their health centers and trained the village health workers, traditional birth attendants, and model mothers. The health centers were all supplied and equipped. A well-child care flipchart was developed to be used for health education in the clinics.

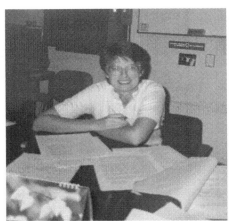

Writing a proposal at my desk in the MOH.

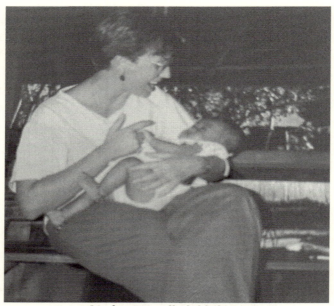
Linda at a well-child clinic.

At the end of the pilot, I visited both the experimental and control health centers with my colleagues. Visiting the control sites was such a contrast to the experimental sites. What a difference! The experimental sites were so popular! Women were walking miles from surrounding villages to the experimental health centers. They were being provided group health education, children received a physical assessment, eye exams, hearing tests, and were given immunizations. The mothers were given individual counseling around their child's growth charts and nutritional status. Mothers received a health card to keep and to bring with them in their return visits. We learned the mothers highly valued these cards, kept them in secure places in their homes, and remembered to bring the cards with them on return visits.

In the final evaluation, the FHD wrote that the pilot project overall appeared to be very successful. The number of well-child care services had increased and the quality of services had greatly improved. More children were being provided comprehensive well-child care services. The mothers were becoming more knowledgeable in their child's care. The FHD recognized it was difficult to measure the impact of this program due to the length of this project and the multiple variables involved. However, with the improvement of the AMWS providing well- child care, they felt it was reasonable to infer that in time the program would help reduce the infant mortality rate, reduce the morbidity of children, and help to decrease the prevalence of malnutrition.

An indicator of the success of the program was when the Director General of the Health Department wanted to start planning for the expansion of the program. I was asked to write another proposal to expand and institutionalize the well-child care services. The University of Michigan agreed to extend my program for nine months. With my supervisors in the Family Health Division, I wrote another proposal which Redd Barna Save the Children agreed to fund. It included incorporating the training curriculum and training materials used in the Maternal Child Centers into the Auxiliary Midwifery Colleges. The colleges would use the thirty-six model well-child clinics for their students practical training. In this way, all future midwifery students would be properly trained in how to provide comprehensive well-child care.

After I left the country, I learned from Thai colleagues that the FHD carried on with this program. I believe the project was successful and sustainable because the government had assessed and identified the need to promote maternal and child health by improving well-child clinics.

Additional Work Experience: Cervical Cancer Screening and HIV Prevention

During my extended stay, the Family Health division asked me to help address cervical cancer, which had been identified as a major public health problem. I used the same strategy as I did for designing the well-child care project; secured funding to organize a conference with all the key gynecologists, pathologists, and cytologists to discuss the problem and design a program.

Prior to the conference, I visited some key hospital labs to assess their capacity to screen and read pap smears. I was shocked to see that many of the cytologists were losing their eyesight due to the large number of slides they screened each day. I also learned that there were only one or two pathologists in the country because many had gone to the United States to work. At the conference, it was determined the Ministry of Health needed to train more cytologists, but meanwhile would pilot the screening with pap smears in a few health centers. I later learned that the Thai government expanded cervical cancer screening.

During my time in Thailand, HIV/AIDs was being recognized as a public health issue. I met people working for organizations who were trying to prevent the spread of the disease by providing education and promoting condoms in the red-light districts of Bangkok. I wanted to learn more so they took me to a bar to talk to some sex workers whom I really enjoyed meeting. I learned more about sex workers when traveling with my co-workers. They took me to one community where they pointed out some large beautiful homes which were funded by the families' daughters who were sex workers. They told me there was no community shame and in fact, families celebrated the birth of a daughter.

Lessons Learned

This internship was an invaluable experience. I learned that my role as an expatriate in Thailand was to assist the Family Health Division of the Ministry of Health to meet their goals and objectives. In order to do this, I had to learn from listening to my Thai colleagues about their health care system, the different cadres of health care workers, their roles and responsibilities, how they were trained and supervised. I learned to use the Thai professionals in the field to set standards, define the roles of the health care workers, write training curriculums, determine the supplies and equipment necessary, and develop health records. As a result of learning from my colleagues and experts in the field, I was able to write proposals, secure funding, and work as a team member in the design, implementation, and evaluation of the project.

I felt a lot of ownership of the project, but I was advised by an experienced and respected expat colleague to always remember that I was working for the Thai government and that all credits, written or verbal, were to go to the Thai government. I followed that advice in all the countries where I later worked. I found working as a facilitator and a team player led to respecting one another which then led to cooperation and collaboration with colleagues essential for a successful and sustainable project.

Even though I didn't take credit for my work, I was honored by a plaque given to me by the Director General of the Department of Health that said, "In recognition of your outstanding contribution to the maternal and child health care training project of the Family Health Division...." I also received a framed appreciation letter from the staff of the Family Health division.

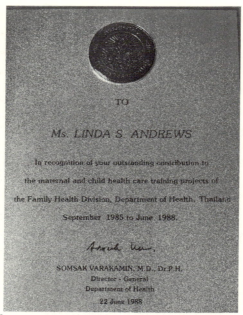

Plaque given to me by the Ministry of Health.

Just before I left Thailand, I was also honored when Tassanee and Dang, my Thai colleagues, gave me a gold ring with my name engraved on it so I wouldn't forget the "Three Musketeers." I wore that ring until 2017, when the ring had to be cut off due to an upcoming surgery.

Exploring Thailand and Celebrating Thai Holidays

Besides my work experience, I had many rich adventures. I was invited by my Thai friends to many wonderful festivals. I was taken to Songkran, a water festival in April which marks the beginning of the traditional Thai New Year. As part of this festival, cleaning images of Buddha was done as well as pouring water on each other representing purification and washing away one's sins.

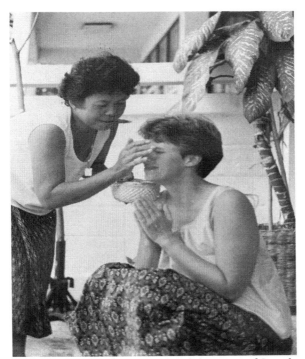

Washing my face with water in celebration of Songkran.

I was in Bangkok on the King's sixtieth birthday and was fortunate to observe a very rare event: the Royal Barge Procession. It was held on the Chao Phraya River which was cleaned of trash for the celebration. There were fifty-three barges going to Wat Arun for a Buddhist ceremony. The king and prince were in one of the boats. There was ancient chanting as the men rowed the barges. All the Thais knew the song, which they learned in school, and they also knew the names of all the barges.

I also observed on the King's birthday, men being offered and given free vasectomies. The goal being to provide this service to 1,000 or more men! It was run by the Thai Population and Community Development Association. The director of the group was Mechai Viravidya. Mechai is known throughout Thailand and worldwide among those working in the field of family planning and HIV/AIDs prevention. He was particularly known for destigmatizing the use of condoms, which were sometimes called mechais. I ate in his restaurant in Bangkok called Cabbages and Condoms.

With my Thai friends, I visited the Karen Hill Tribe in the north, along the Myanmar-Thailand border. They are refugees from Burma with elongated necks and wore heavy brass rings around their necks, forearms, and shins. I also visited the golden triangle, the area where the borders of Thailand, Laos, and Myanmar (formerly Burma) meet at the confluence of the Ruak and Mekong rivers.

I was fascinated when my colleagues took me to see a soccer game played by one hundred elephants. Many of the elephants are domesticated, and some of the elephant keepers, called mahouts, train their elephants to play soccer called football. It was quite an exciting experience!

Exploring Outside Thailand

I was able to see some of the surrounding countries with my American Peace Corps friends. The most memorable trip was a week touring Myanmar. The country was tightly controlled by the government and restricted in terms of how long you stayed and where you could travel. I was able to explore Rangoon (Yangon) and see many pagodas. I flew in a rickety plane to Inle Lake, where I canoed around the floating vegetable gardens and saw men using their feet to paddle their boat. We went to Pagan to see Buddhist pagodas and to canoe down the Irrawaddy River. There were no cars in Pagan, only bicycles and horses. I remember a lovely moonlight ride to a restaurant in a horse-driven cart. We traveled to Mandalay and sat on the steps of the Mandalay Palace. It was an amazing trip.

I took another trip, with the same Peace Corps friends, to explore Hong Kong and to visit some of the smaller islands not far from the mainland. I feel very fortunate in having all these amazing opportunities!

Decision to Continue My International Career

I admit the first year was emotionally rocky while learning to overcome culture shock and figuring out my role as an intern within the Ministry of Health. However, at no point did I doubt that I wanted to continue working in international health.
I am so grateful that I persevered to realize my dream. I got to experience the Thai culture first-hand and I learned something new every day! I loved working with my Thai colleagues and I feel so grateful they accepted me and helped me to understand and cross any cultural barriers. At age forty, I finally had all the credentials needed to proceed in my career in international health.

Somalia
September 1988-October 1990

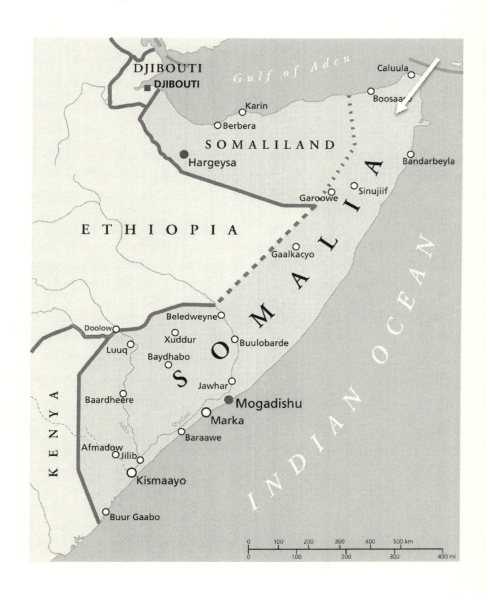

Finding My Next Position and Settling In

After more than three years, my contract in Thailand was ending, and as luck would have it, a friend told me about a two-year position in Somalia with a U.S. contractor. This position was a part of a USAID-funded Family Health Services (FHS) project. They were looking for a technical advisor to work with the Somali Family Health/Family Planning (FH/FP) Division of the Ministry of Health. A friend had worked there and encouraged me with stories of the exotic environment, friendly people, and a government eager to advance work on women's health. I applied and was accepted!

When I flew over Somalia in September of 1988, I saw for the first time a semi-desert land, sparsely populated, with vast expanses of long, sandy, desolate beaches. I wondered if I had made a big mistake by accepting this position; what a contrast to the tropical paradise of Thailand!

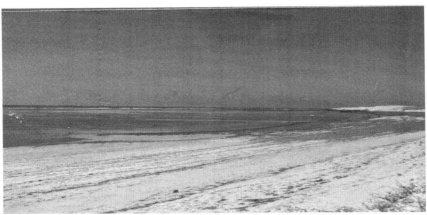

Typical desolate beaches outside Mogadishu.

Again, I would have to overcome many of the same challenges as in Thailand; I had to create a home, learn how to get around, adapt to new foods, learn some Arabic, make friends, and learn how to live and work in a new culture. Communication with my family would be even more limited than in Thailand; because there were no telephones, I had to rely solely on handwritten letters.

I was fortunate my new employer already had arranged a beautifully furnished house for me. It was located in the capital, Mogadishu. It had a great deck and a large backyard with a resident tortoise. My house was surrounded by a cement wall topped with circular barbed wire, barred windows, and I had a twenty-four-hour guard service. The U.S. Embassy issued me a hand-held radio to use in case of an emergency. Every morning I was called by the U.S. Marines to ensure that the radio was working.

I was provided a Jeep and driver to use for work. It was necessary to have four-wheel drive in case I got stuck in the sand. I had to be trained how to get into four-wheel drive, which involved getting out of the Jeep and changing it manually!

Expats were expected to employ cooks, gardeners, guards, etc. This was seen as a great employment opportunity for locals and third country nationals. I hired a young Ethiopian woman as my cook, who introduced me to her native cuisine. I had never seen or eaten injera, a fermented pancake-like flatbread. I had to ask her how to eat it! (I now love Ethiopian food!) I wanted to celebrate Thanksgiving by sharing a turkey I had shipped in from Kenya with my Somali colleagues. However, when I invited them, they explained they preferred goat; they had eaten turkey before and said it was too dry! My cook then made a delicious Thanksgiving meal of goat over an open fire in my backyard. I later roasted and shared the turkey with my expat friends with my cook watching me, eager to learn!

I enjoyed the local foods. Sometimes on the weekends, I would be invited to go with the Somali nurses to eat lunch at a local "bush" restaurant, which served roasted baby goat with rice and a special spiced sauce. We would sit on a large mat under an acacia tree, eating with our fingers from one large platter. It was delicious!

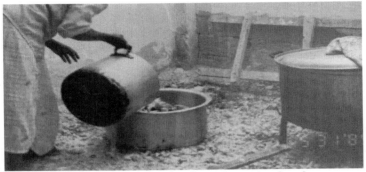

In my backyard cooking goat for Thanksgiving using local common pots.

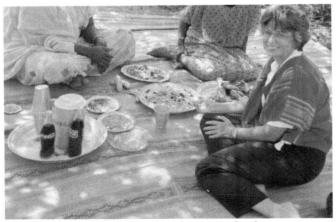

Sharing a platter of goat/veg/rice at a bush restaurant.

There also were restaurants that served fresh seafood including large, naturally sweet lobsters, no butter needed! You could even buy cappuccinos because of the historical influence of the Italians.

I felt more accepted by the Somali people when I wore their traditional attire, a long one-piece dress with a long scarf that could cover your head and drape over the shoulders. It was very comfortable to wear in the heat and you could use the scarf to protect your head and face from the sun and sand. I found some beautiful cotton African prints that I had sewn into traditional one-piece full-length dresses and I bought colorful scarves to go with it.

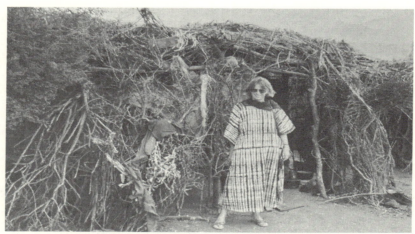

In local dress in front of a tea house in Mogadishu.

I didn't cover my head as did the Somali women. Since they were Muslim and it was a part of their culture/religion, they did not expect me, as a Christian, to cover my head.

Somalia was known in East Africa for their henna and designs. I joined the nurses to have elaborate henna designs drawn on my hands, forearms, and feet. We would sit for hours outdoors in the shade as the henna was applied and dried. When you removed the dried paste, it left intricate designs that lasted for weeks.

I didn't know anyone upon arriving, but made friends easily. The Somali nurses and doctors were warm and welcoming, I felt a part of the team immediately. I was taken into their homes and was invited to their family celebrations, took part in their birthing rituals, and funerals. There was a small community of expats from many different countries and I made friends with people from England, Ireland, Norway, and Germany. Since the U.S. had a military base there, I also made some very good friends among the Army and Navy personnel.

In my first year, I enjoyed living and working in Mogadishu and felt safe driving and walking around the town; it was so peaceful at night with the bright stars and the sound of the ocean. However, in my second year, a Somali civil war spread throughout the country. The President, Mohamed Siad Barre, had ruled the Muslim country for twenty-one years, but now the country had split into warring clans. Driving in and outside of Mogadishu was no longer safe due to roadblocks by men with AK-47s, kids with hand grenades, and frequent sounds of explosions. Eventually, we had a curfew because it was too dangerous to go out at night. My contract ended in October 1990 and I left the country just as the violence was escalating in Mogadishu.

Work Experience

The Family Health/Family Planning (FH/FP) office was a one-story cement building which had barred open windows with shutters that locked. I remember it being very dry and dusty due to the semi-desert environment. Some days it was just too hot to work in the office, so we would work out of my house which had air-conditioning.

An interesting challenge of my work in Somalia was the advent of computer technology. After years of writing manually-typed reports, I now was expected to submit reports using a computer. But first, I had to learn how to use it! I had the usual technology disasters; one being not backing up my work and losing the newly-developed curriculum. Thank heavens I had a hard copy, which then had to be entirely reentered into the computer.

For two years I had a wonderful nurse counterpart, whom I will refer to as H.S. She and I worked closely together and became good friends. She was serious about her work, respected by the staff and, fortunately for me, fluent in English. H.S. not only worked full time with the FH/FP division, but also worked with the feminist political party called SWDO (Somali Women's Democratic Organization). This organization was fighting the practice of female circumcision.

As my counterpart, H.S. helped me to navigate the Somali culture. One of my biggest adjustments was switching from the non-confrontational Thai culture to a culture that was confrontational. After one very argumentative meeting with raised voices, H.S. saw that I was very upset and took me aside and explained this was their normal way of behavior and not to worry.

My position as the long-term advisor was to work with the Somali doctors and nurses to assist in improving and increasing FP/FH services. There was as a pervasive negative cultural attitude about limiting family size, therefore, we focused on using contraception to space the children two to three years apart. Particularly in developing countries, this gives mothers time to recover from her last pregnancy and be ready for her next pregnancy. In Somalia, the most acceptable method of spacing children was exclusive breastfeeding for the first six months postpartum. There is a high degree of contraceptive protection during lactational amenorrhea (no menses while breastfeeding), but after the menses returned, another form of contraceptive was advised.

Modern birth control methods were not widely used, even though the nurses and doctors were trained in all methods. Many of the FH/FP nurses were trained in IUD insertions in Kenya because IUDs were more accepted there and they could get sufficient clinical practice. Condoms became a big part of the family planning campaign due to concerns about the new spread of HIV/AIDS.

In light of the cultural attitudes, we were able to work effectively as a team and accomplished a lot together. Our major achievement was developing a FH/FP training manual for health professionals in English and a reference manual in Somali.

There were few printed health educational materials. In the classrooms, everything was written on flipcharts and the different contraceptive methods were demonstrated.

We trained tutors in the midwifery schools and incorporated FH/FP into the school's curriculum. We trained health care workers, traditional birth attendants, and villagers.

To be sure the hospitals and health centers did not run out of their supply of contraceptives, we developed a logistic system to manage the ordering and supplying of contraceptives. Ordering was a challenge because the contraceptives were purchased and imported by different international organizations and this involved a lot of coordination.

Another very significant accomplishment was adding to the family planning clinic in the main hospital in Mogadishu, the service of diagnosing and treating sexually transmitted infections (STIs). The nurses and doctors were trained to diagnose with the use of a microscope which our project imported with all the related necessary supplies. The clinicians were extremely eager and grateful to learn; it was clearly an unmet need for many women who suffered with STIs.

I think it was due to the popularity of this clinic that an elderly man saw this as an opportunity to earn money. One day I was going to observe the clinic when I found this man had roped off the stairwell to the clinic. He was asking for money to go upstairs! I could not believe it! This was addressed with the hospital administration and was stopped.

To accomplish the above, I used the same lessons I learned in Thailand, which was to listen and learn from my Somali colleagues and to work as a team member. As in Thailand, I developed close personal friendships in the FH/FP division which built trust and respect for each other and made the work fun which is so important in achieving goals and objectives. When I returned to the United States, I was honored by receiving the annual technical assistance award from my contracting agency.

Sadly, two months after I left the country, the violence escalated among the clans and the government collapsed. I do not know what happened to my colleagues and all that we accomplished. I only hope they are safe and that somehow what was learned was beneficial to their lives and others.

Female Circumcision

Even though my focus within the FH/FP Division was family planning, a major women's health issue was female circumcision. The nurses I worked with knew very well the side effects and complications of circumcision. When we went to the villages to provide family planning education, they would take this opportunity to discuss these dangers and a safe alternative to circumcision. They were also active members of SWDO.

Most women in Somalia were circumcised. It usually happened when a girl was between the ages of five and nine. It is not a religious obligation, instead it is carried out to ensure virginity and it is tied to family honor. At this time, it was mainly a ritual performed by local women using knives, scissors, or razor blades that were not disinfected and without anesthesia. There are different forms of female circumcision, but the most common type in Somalia was Type III, the most harmful type. "It is the removal of part or all of the external genitalia [clitoris, labia minora and labia majora] and stitching the vaginal opening, leaving a very small opening, about the size of a matchstick, to allow for the flow of urine and menstrual blood."[2] I will never forget when I was shown a very long, sharp thorn of a tree that was used for stitching the vaginal opening.

---

[2] https://2001-2009.state.gov/g/wi/rls/rep/crfgm/index.htm

I learned a lot from the nurses I worked with and from the members of SWDO. They explained to me that when women have intercourse for the first time, it is very painful and many women bleed from the tearing. This bleeding is seen as a positive sign by the husband and family for it means that she has not been with other men.

Female circumcision can cause many problems. There are the immediate problems after cutting such as pain, bleeding, infections such as tetanus, urinary problems, and some women even die. There are many long-term complications such as urinary and vaginal infections, menstrual problems, complications during childbirth, and increased risk of newborn deaths.

One major complication of childbirth that could occur with unmanaged prolonged labor was the development of a vaginal or rectal fistula. With the baby's head unable to get through the vaginal opening, the head presses against the wall of the vagina and can cause a fistula or abnormal opening between the vagina and bladder and/or the vagina and rectum. An opening between the vagina and bladder causes women to leak urine. An opening between the vagina and rectum causes the leaking of feces. With both types of fistulas, woman may have a very bad odor, which usually leads to being ostracized from her community. These fistulas can be repaired by surgery, but it is not an easy procedure. When I was there, specialized doctors were brought to Somalia to do repairs.

My colleagues taught that you could substitute female circumcision with a symbolic procedure which was having a knife just prick the skin of the genitalia. Liberal imams in Saudi Arabia supported this substitution and were invited to come to Somalia to advocate for it.

On one memorable field trip, I traveled with eight Somali women to teach villagers about family planning and to discuss female circumcision. As we were driving, three of the women told me about their circumcisions. I kept a journal of the stories that I heard and these are my edited notes from 1988 to 1990. I will address them as Colleagues 1, 2, and 3.

Colleague 1: She was seven or eight years old when she was circumcised. They told her it wouldn't hurt, be like a feather. Two women came and held her down and she was blindfolded. They used knives, no anesthesia. When she screamed, they beat drums so no one could hear her. She was in great pain, for fourteen days she didn't urinate. She bled a great deal, there was a lot of pus. She said she was lucky to be alive today. She never knew you were supposed to have one opening for urination and another one for menstruation. They cut off her clitoris and some parts of the labia and then sewed the remaining labia, leaving one opening for both urine and menses.

Colleague 2: Her mother didn't believe in female circumcision and didn't want her daughter to be circumcised. Her grandmother disagreed, wailed, and walked out of the house. Due to her grandmother's insistence, she cried, "Mom, I want to be circumcised" She was eight years old. She was circumcised. Her mother cried. The daughter now regrets her decision. However, she still has part of her clitoris.

Colleague 3: She was circumcised at five years old. She explained after circumcision, you sat over a dug-out hole in the ground with wood steam to dry the incision. This hole was attached to another hole with burning charcoal. You blew over one and the heat went up the other. She did not circumcise her own daughter.

I was also told that some of the FH/FP staff, who went to Kenya for IUD insertion training, saw for the first-time women who were not circumcised. One Kenyan patient requested the Somali trainee to not touch her clitoris because it was sensitive. The trainee did not understand because she was circumcised so another trainee had to explain to her why.

My only contribution to the discussion of female circumcision occurred one Sunday afternoon eating at a bush restaurant with H.S. and two of her friends. After we had a delicious meal, sharing one large platter of roasted goat, we lay down to talk and rest. H.S. told me that one of her friends still had a clitoris and would I explain to her about the clitoris and orgasms. It took me by surprise, but I was honored that H.S. felt comfortable to ask me. The friend was eager to learn, so I explained the best I could. I didn't see this woman again for several months, then one day, when I was at a buffet dinner with my Somali friends, she came up to me with a big smile on her face, and then we both smiled knowingly. I later learned her mother protected her from being circumcised, but she was still having a lot of pressure from her grandmother to be circumcised.

Learning About Cultural Practices Around Childbirth

It really is a privilege to learn about and experience other cultural practices first-hand. Because of the high infant mortality rate, families didn't name or celebrate their child's birth until the child was a year old. I learned not to ask what the baby's name was until after the one-year birthday and that most Somalis don't celebrate birthdays because there are too many children and they do not have a lot of money.

However, H.S. did take me to a birthday party for a one-year-old. There were only women at the party and we all sat on the floor facing a table with a cake on it. There was incense and music from a boom box. The child cut the cake and someone gave the child a bite and we all sang "Happy Birthday." The city power had gone off, so they used candles and kerosene burners. After cutting the cake, we all danced to Somali music. I had on a Somali dress so while dancing, H.S. wrapped a large scarf around my hips and showed me how to dance using my hips African-style. I had a great time trying to imitate their movements!

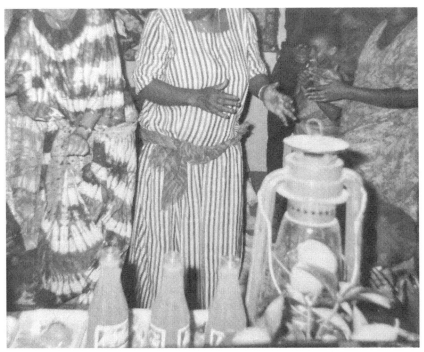

Learning to dance using a scarf tied around my hips.

Somali women were really afraid of dying in childbirth, as the maternal mortality was very high. It was predicted then that

2,600 women would die that year due to maternal-related cases. H.S. invited me one afternoon to a traditional ceremony to pray for a woman, who was almost nine months pregnant, to have a safe delivery. I entered a room of ten to fifteen women sitting on the floor in a circle on mats. The expectant woman served us rice and goat on a large platter with a banana and a plate of salad. As was the custom, we all ate with our fingers. We were also served a delicious goat soup served in a glass. We had lemon juice to drink and watermelon and papaya for dessert.

After the meal, the expectant woman sat in the middle of the circle. An elder woman chanted prayers and we all repeated her chant. She would pray for two to three sentences and we would chant back. Sometimes we clapped to the chants. We all raised our hands up to pray. Then we reached out toward the expectant mother and chanted. She reached out and held our hands. We were all focused on her and prayed her delivery would be as "easy as a cat vomits." Each person placed their scarf/veil over their head and held a container of myrrh under the veil. The scent was to get in your hair and clothes. Two different kinds of perfume were then put on each of us. We continually prayed. Afterwards we had popcorn and Somali tea. It was a wonderful experience.

Self-Entertainment

I love seeing and learning about the African wildlife! Besides the large tortoise in my backyard, it was the camels that fascinated me. I loved watching them and their young. They were so prevalent just outside of Mogadishu. These camels were not ridden, but used as pack animals and a source of milk and meat. I loved watching the nomads with their bright, colorful, flowing robes walking along with their camels which were packed with their household goods. We would watch the camels drink at the watering holes. One day, I saw the nomads collect the camel's urine in buckets. I was told the urine was poured over the sheep to treat them for skin diseases. I do not know if this was true or not but it was an interesting explanation. There were also many donkeys pulling carts with goods. I felt like I was living in Biblical times!

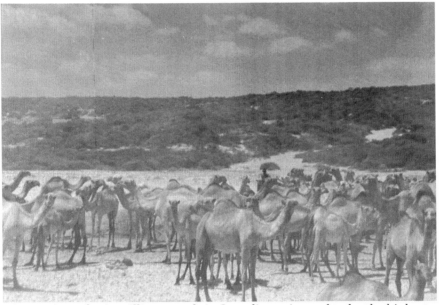

Approximately six million camels in Somalia, estimated to be the highest number per country in 2023. Most are used as pack animals.

I am always entertained by birdwatching. I met some Canadians who took me to a salt lake not far from Mogadishu. The lake was amidst sand dunes, no trees, but there were shrubs around the lake. In the lake we saw lots and lots of flamingos! I was also taken to Balcad Nature Reserve, a riverine forest along the Shebelle River. It was established by the Somali Ecological Society in 1985. I often went to this reserve to birdwatch and see the monkeys. One day, a friend, who was a British veterinarian, went walking in the reserve and accidentally disturbed a bee's hive. They swarmed her and she had to make a choice whether to be stung or to jump in the river filled with crocodiles and hippos! She decided to jump in the river and luckily, she survived. After this, I was more cautious birdwatching!

I loved to play on the sandy beaches and soak in the pools in the rocks, but did not swim. The ocean around Mogadishu was infested with Zambezi River sharks. They were attracted to the smell of camel intestines dumped into the sea by city butchers. The sharks would come close to the shore so you couldn't even play in the waves or sit in the ocean. Before I arrived in Somalia, I heard one young expat girl was killed on the beach and one person lost her leg sitting in the water.

There was no lack of a social life. The U.S. military had a base in Somalia and many of the military men were housed in Mogadishu. They provided the whole expat community with lots of fun. They were from the Marine corps, Army, and Navy branches. I was privileged to be invited to the annual American Marine Ball by the gunny (gunnery) sergeant, a top-ranking Marine, and one of the few men who was single. Many of the guys loved to go fishing and would invite the community for great barbecues. I think it was the first time I had fresh tuna. On weekends, the expats would caravan out to the remote pristine beaches for picnics. I usually traveled with my military friends because I felt safe and secure with their skills driving in the desert. We did crazy things like driving up and down sand dunes and we did this until we learned that murdered bodies maybe hidden in some of these dunes! The military vehicles were equipped with winches; if any car got stuck on the beach, they were able to winch it out before the tide came in and destroyed the vehicle. They winched many cars that got stranded on the beach!

There was also an international school in Mogadishu and I made good friends with many of the American teachers. One of them had rescued a giant eagle owl. When out of its cage, the owl would jump up and look in the windows of the classroom. The students raised mice to feed the owl and one summer it was my duty to feed the owl. I got dead mice and had to climb into the cage to feed it. When the country was collapsing, a pilot, in his small plane, flew the owl to Kenya for safety!

Other activities included dancing, volleyball, and running in the semi desert. I met a United Nations pilot from Venezuela, who taught salsa and meringue. I became his main dance partner and we danced every party we could.

Traveling Outside Somalia

Since Somalia bordered Kenya to the south, I often visited and toured the country. I would fly every few months to Nairobi for a haircut. I also spent time exploring Kenya with my best friend, Pat, visiting from Washington State. We went on a safari in Maasai Mara National Reserve, snorkeled on a famous reef near Malindi, and sailed on a dhow (wooden sailboat) off of Lamu Island. The town of Lamu was fascinating. It was founded in the twelve century and is an educational center for Islamic and Swahili culture. We also traveled from Nairobi to Mombasa on an old colonial train which was really a unique experience.

Leaving Somalia was Traumatic

One weekend near the end of my contract, I didn't go to the beach with my expatriate friends, but instead stayed back to finish up some work. I was so glad I didn't go; they were ambushed by a group of Somali men with AK-47s who sprayed them with bullets. They ran and hid behind their cars and fortunately no one was killed. After that incident, no one ever went to the beach again. It was also too dangerous to even travel on the road to the beaches because there were illegal roadblocks where cars were stopped and robbed.

Several months before I left Mogadishu, I began to hear gunshots and grenades exploding. Road blocks by Somali soldiers began to appear in the city. I had to be careful going to and from work. It was good that I usually traveled with the Somali nurses who were able to get me through the roadblocks. I started carrying my radio so I could alert the U.S. Embassy of issues and they could alert me of dangerous areas. In fact, all the expats started carrying their radios. When I had dinner with my expat friends from different countries and organizations, we would put our radios in front of us on the table. When we heard an explosion, we would share with each other what information was known and report in to our organizations.

Two weeks before I was to leave Somalia, I packed up my house and moved to a guesthouse, where I was the only one staying except for a cook who was there during the day. I checked out the security. There was a cement wall around the guesthouse with a guard by the gate entrance. The guard made a hole in the gate so he could see who wanted to come into the guesthouse grounds. I gave the guard a whistle so that he could warn me if anyone tried to enter. One early morning, there were gunshots outside the guesthouse. I was scared and called the Marines on the radio. They could only give me one piece of advice—to not go near the window. I lay in bed wondering what was happening. Finally, the cook came to prepare breakfast and told me that some robbers were stealing copper wires from next door and the guards were shooting.

I was fortunate my contract ended in mid-October 1990. The country was becoming too dangerous to live in and it was a scary time. Many expats left, but some stayed on too long and had to fly out before they could pack and ship their household goods. With too little time, some packed their personal and household belongings in containers and stored them within the walls of the U.S. Embassy compound. On January 1, the Somalis climbed over the U.S. embassy wall and pillaged the compound. The U.S. ambassador and a few staff were rescued by helicopter.

I learned a very important lesson: countries can quickly turn into dangerous places!

Bangladesh
April 1991–October 1995

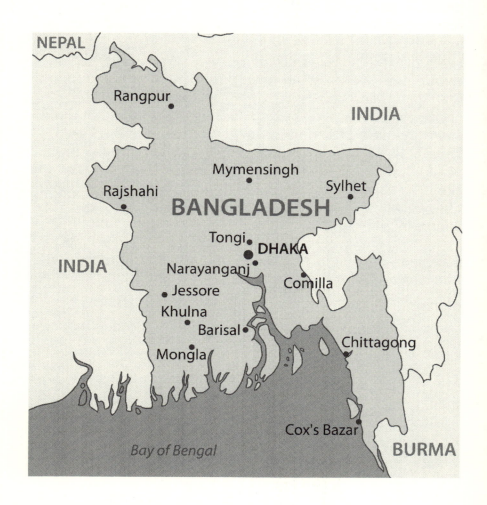

Finding a Job and Settling In

One afternoon in September of 1990, in a little cafeteria in
Mogadishu, I encountered an American friend who informed

me of a USAID job opening in Bangladesh. It was a position as a Clinical Services Program Manager working in the USAID Population and Health office. I would be employed under a personal service contract (PSC). I applied, was flown to Bangladesh for an extensive interview including field trips, and was accepted for the position. This would be my first personal service contract with USAID. I went on to work as a PSC with USAID for a total of twelve years: four years in Bangladesh, two years in Kazakhstan, and five years in Malawi.

My Somali contract ended in October 1990. However, due to the Gulf War, I couldn't start my new position immediately. I returned to the U.S. and waited almost five months for the war to end. In late March of 1991, the USAID office in Bangladesh decided it was safe for me to travel. I was delayed enroute because of some documents that had not yet been signed, so I spent time with friends in London and in Stavanger, Norway. These were friends I had worked with in Somalia, so it was a fun reunion. I finally arrived in Dhaka just before my forty-fourth birthday, April 25.

By far, Bangladesh was safer to live in than Somalia, but I had never seen such an over-populated country with extreme poverty. When driving in the capital of Dhaka, it was shocking to see malnourished mothers with their babies, and crippled men, women, and children in the median strip of a two-way highway begging for money. On side streets, I saw men who couldn't walk and got around by lying on boards with wheels and pushing themselves with their arms. I saw people who just rolled their bodies to get around. It was heartbreaking.

Settling in Dhaka was much easier than in other countries since I was working with other Americans in the USAID office. The only hard part was finding my own home. I was lucky to find a lovely two-story home with an outdoor deck in a clean and quiet area called Baridhara. I had about the same security measures as when I worked in Somalia, a secure wall around the compound with security lights, barred windows, panic buttons inside the house and a 24-hour guard. I did have a landline phone which I did not have in Somalia.

I was really fortunate that Alex, a USAID colleague, and Betsy, his wife, lived a short walking distance from my house. They were incredibly warm and welcoming. I later met and began dating Bob, a Canadian, who was working for an American international organization. Bob and I were invited to all of Alex and Betsy's weekly badminton tournaments, where we met many more people. We celebrated all the holidays together at which Alex hired unusual local talent, including a local snake charmer and street bands. Betsy and Alex also organized interesting and amazing vacations and included the two of us. We went with them to Calcutta, Darjeeling, Sikkim, Bhutan, and Nepal.

The USAID office was located in the suburbs of Dhaka in a new large red brick building that included both USAID and the U.S. Embassy. It looked like a fort and was well guarded by U.S. marines and since I had just come from Somalia, this gave me peace of mind. For transportation, I purchased a second-hand Subaru that had been imported from the U.S. It was a fine car, but the steering wheel was on the right side of the car. In Bangladesh, you drove on the left side of the road. It was a bit tricky when trying to pass a vehicle because it was difficult to see around the car in front of you since you were sitting on the shoulder side of the road! I would use a bicycle rickshaw to get around when possible. I enjoyed taking rickshaws, especially in the evening when the moon was full! I had my favorite rickshaw wallas (drivers) whom I trusted to take me to nearby events. They would wait for me and bring me home safely.

Work Experience

My original job description was to work with the Family Planning and Family Health Division of the Ministry of Health to improve the contraceptive prevalence rate by increasing access to family planning services through satellite (rural) health clinics. The Bangladesh Demographic Health Survey (DHS) of 1993-1994, a survey funded by USAID every 5 years, reported the contraceptive prevalence rate was 44.6% of the currently married women age 10-49. Of the temporary methods, 17.4 % used oral contraceptives pills, 4.5% injectables, 3% condoms and 2.2% IUDs (Intrauterine devices). Traditional method use was 8.4% and 9.2 % sterilization.

However, after observing health care workers providing FP services in the health centers with the government and non-governmental organizations (NGOs), it was determined there was a need to focus on improving the quality and availability of clinical family planning services. Clinical services included the provision of the IUDs which was the Copper 7, and injectable contraceptive methods which included Depo-Provera, a three-month injectable, and Net-EN, a two-month injectable.

In the first months, I met the key government players in the provision of family planning services. In the Ministry of Health, I met with the Project Director of Clinical Services with whom I would be working closely and to whom I would report. I also met with counterparts from the National Institute for Population Research and training (NIPORT). This is the institute which provided the basic training for the Family Welfare Workers (FWVs) who provided the clinical services. I was introduced to the Family Planning Clinical Supervisory Team (FPCST). This was a team of government physicians that conducted supervisory visits in the health facilities and provided refresher training to the Family Welfare Workers and the physicians providing FP clinical services.

I was also given a formal introduction and orientation to three key USAID funded NGOs who worked in partnership with the government in the provision of family planning. These included (1) The Association for Voluntary Surgical Contraception (AVSC), now called EngenderHealth; (2) The Asia Foundation; and (3) The Johns Hopkins Center for Communication Programs. Another NGO partner was the Rural MCH-FP Extension Project of the International Center for Diarrhea Disease Research in Bangladesh (ICDDR, B).

I developed very good working relationships with all the partners and worked as a team member to improve the quality and availability of family planning services. Together we traveled to many health centers to observe their practices, identify issues, and with health care providers, work out solutions.

Improving the Quality and Availability of IUD Services

The main concerns with the practice of inserting an IUD was (1) Not using the proper technique for insertion; (2) Not using proper infection prevention techniques; and (3) Not knowing how to manage clients with side effects.

The quality of IUD services was addressed by the following:

1. Improved the training of the health care providers by developing national guidelines for FP clinical services, a training manual and materials for service provider's basic and refresher training.

2. Developed a national standardized list of furniture, equipment, and supplies necessary for inserting an IUD.

3. Developed an IUD insertion training video. Even though we had support from an international NGO with expertise in video production, it took a lot of time and effort in writing a script, selecting local actors, setting the proper stage, filming, and then editing. In addition to the training video, a locally made pelvic model was developed by AVSC in order for providers to practice their pelvic exams and IUD insertions. The few models available were very expensive ones imported from the U.S.

4. Introduced a new procedure called decontamination, this was placing used instruments and exam gloves directly into a bucket of .5 percent chlorine solution for 10 minutes. This kills any viruses including HIV and bacteria to make them safe to clean. This involved purchasing buckets and chlorine and training health care staff to make the .5 percent chlorine solution. This also included purchasing and using utility gloves instead of using bare hands to wash and rinse instruments and gloves after decontamination.

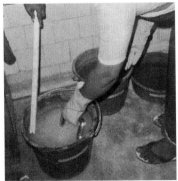

Decontamination of used instruments.

5. Adapted a portable steam sterilizer that could sterilize three sets of IUD instruments including gloves and cotton balls. The steam sterilizer was found in most health centers for they had been used to sterilize glass syringes before the introduction of disposable syringes and needles. This method of sterilizing IUD instruments was tested and approved by PATH (Program of Appropriate Technology in Health) and was written up in the American Journal of Infection Control.[3]

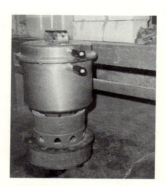

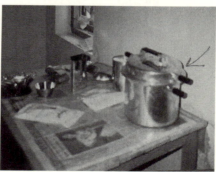

IUD instrument steam sterilizer contains three sets
of instruments, cotton balls, and gloves.

---

[3] Mark Barone et al, American Journal of Infection Control, August 1997, Practice Forum Adaptation and validation of a portable steam sterilizer for processing intrauterine device insertion instruments and supplies in low resource settings, August 1997, pages 350-356, 17/49/81108

6. Availability was improved by designing and making backpacks for the portable sterilizer. I had fun traveling by rickshaw to homes and piloting home insertions.

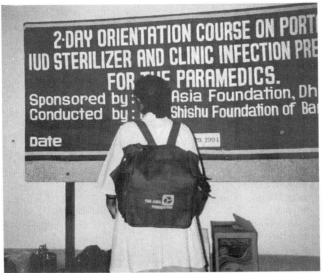

Backpack with portable IUD instrument steam sterilizer.

Prior to my leaving, 87 NGOs were using the IUD instrument sterilizers and the Bangladesh government approved the sterilizer and allotted funds to purchase 6,000 sterilizers with a backpack and timer for all the FP clinics.

7. Formed a medical advisory committee and developed National Guidelines for treatment of sexually transmitted diseases (STIs) and pelvic inflammatory disease (PID). There was a new protocol for treatment which was based on symptoms not lab results using microscopes. This was called syndromic management. With syndromic management, identification and treatment could be done at the rural level.

After approval of the guidelines, the government ordered and distributed the appropriate drugs and sent out a circular regarding the proper treatment of PID and STIs. Health care trainers, government medical supervisors, and medical officers from non-governmental organizations were oriented.

Improving the Quality of Contraceptive Injectable Services

The main concern with the administration of the injectable contraceptives was the unsafe handling and disposing of the used disposable syringes and needles. Some health providers were putting the cap back on the needle after using it. This increased the risk of being pricked and being exposed to HIV and hepatitis B or C. The used syringes and needles were seen thrown out the back window of the health center with other trash and children seen playing with them. They also were seen stored in open cardboard boxes under patient benches or mixed in boxes with books, paper, etc.

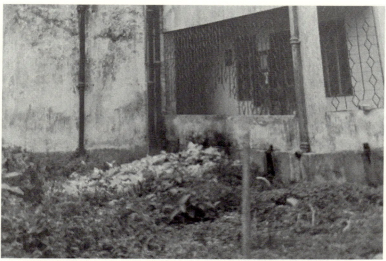

Used syringes and needles thrown outside health center.

The proper disposal of syringes and needles were addressed by the following:

1. Trained health providers to dispose the syringe and uncapped needle directly into a puncture proof, burnable container. This container had to be one that would be difficult for anyone to remove the syringes and needles. (In later years, cardboard containers or plastic containers were provided to health centers for the safe disposal of syringes and needles.)

2. Trained health facility staff how to make or use an existing incinerator to burn the syringes and needles. After burning, the leftover burnt metal needles were to be carefully shoveled into pits and buried.

   During my field visits, I assessed the incinerators that were being built or were already built and the pits for burying the needles. I never imagined I would become so knowledgeable on locally made incinerators!

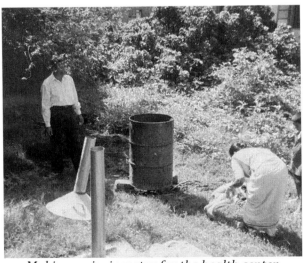

Making an incinerator for the health center.

3. Developed a National Disposal policy and procedures for syringes and needles and the Family Planning Clinical Surveillance team were to monitor the system.

4. Availability was addressed by an NGO that piloted delivering injectables door to door.

After four years working with the government and with the NGOs, we were able to improve the quality and availability of the IUD and injectable services. As a team we were able to identify the key issues that needed to be addressed and then were able to implement the solutions. After my contract had ended, USAID continued funding to build on these accomplishments in order to improve the quality of family planning clinical services.

My USAID supervisor wrote in my final evaluation, "The National Family program, specifically in the area of clinical contraception and quality assurance, has been well served by Ms. Andrews; she was instrumental in helping to put into place many of the essential building blocks for a higher quality and more accessible clinical services program."

Study tour: Indonesia

As part of my job, I was fortunate to be able to go on two short family planning study tours; one in Indonesia and the other in China. I went to Indonesia with my Bangladeshi colleagues to study the management of their national family planning program. Indonesia was well known for its success in delivering family planning services. We spent time visiting health centers on the island of Java, visiting various government and NGO offices in Jakarta, and traveled to the island of Sumatra to observe their health centers. We felt there were lessons learned that we could incorporate in Bangladesh.

Study tour: China

The other trip was a two-week trip to China to study the country's family planning program. This program was organized and attended by American health professionals. The Chinese policy at that time was that each couple could only have one child and the preference was to have a boy.

Prior to the trip, I requested that I be able to observe family planning services in the rural areas. I was taken on a personal tour of a typical village. I was surprised to see how each women's reproductive lives were closely monitored. There were government officials in the village who knew what each woman was using for birth control and when their menses was expected. If they became pregnant, they would usually have an ultrasound to determine the sex of the child. Abortions and adoptions were common if the child was a girl. It was interesting and a little disturbing to see so many families with one child and usually a boy.

I have to mention as part of this study tour, I was able to see and walk on the Great Wall of China!

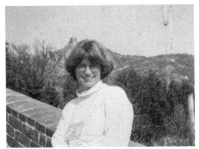

Standing at the Great Wall in China.

Self-Entertainment

Part of living overseas is the ability to create your own entertainment. I was turning forty-five years old and always wanted to be a back-up singer in a rock band. So for my birthday, I gathered the musicians and singers in my social circle and we surprised my guests with a raucous 60s band. We sang four songs and were a hit! We called ourselves "The Committed." We then expanded our song list and played for many rooftop parties. We had an American saxophone player who had played with The Four Tops, a Dutch drummer, a French guitar player, and some excellent singers of all nationalities. Since there were many fabric shops and many local tailors, we outfitted ourselves with amazing glittery outfits! The band's largest attended performance was at the Diarrhea Ball, a fundraiser for the International Center for Diarrhea Disease Research. More than 300 people came to support the ball!

Dancing is a great form of entertainment. I improved my ballroom dancing by taking lessons from a Bangladeshi who offered lessons. He worked for the World Bank and had learned ballroom dancing in Hawaii while getting his Ph.D. His classes were full and very popular. During this time, he taught his new wife to be his dance partner. She did ballroom dancing in a sari! I also learned and taught country western line dancing. With a USAID colleague, we taught ourselves using instructional videos. Once we had memorized the dance steps, we then organized parties to teach others. I could usually find a way to dance to local music and/or international music in every country.

Moonlight boating was a lot of fun. During this time, my friend Alex thought it would be great to buy a local river boat and cruise the Tongi River, a very muddy and polluted river not far outside of Dhaka. Rob, a former UCLA classmate who was interning in the USAID office, thought this was a great idea so together we bought a large, old wooden boat. When the moon was full, an e-mail went out to all our friends who would come and bring guitars for singing and food to share. I understand that now many expats have bought boats and moonlight cruises continue. A lot of business was generated for the local boat men who would sell their boats and then were paid to repair them.

Christmas was a special time. I loved spending Christmas mornings with Mother Teresa's orphanage. Several of my friends and I arrived early in the morning with presents and donated money for a chicken dinner, which was a very special meal for them. We knew the orphans personally because we would frequently organize trips and special events for them. We even organized a boat ride down the Tongi River, which they loved!

Bicycle rickshaw caroling also became a way of celebrating Christmas. This involved hiring and decorating a bicycle rickshaw and then going from house to house for drinks, food, and caroling. Since this is mainly a Muslim country, we selected Christian homes to visit. The rickshaw wallas loved this event due to the fun they had and the money they generated! I have heard that this tradition has continued and the number of hired rickshaws has grown tremendously resulting in needing people to control the traffic!

I became a regular member of the Dhaka Hash which met weekly and was very popular. The Hash is formally called the Hash House Harriers. It was founded in 1938 in Kuala Lumpur by British soldiers and expatriates who started going for weekly runs to shake off their weekend hangovers. This small group evolved into one of the world's biggest running collectives. Hashes are held weekly in almost every major city and can be found online. You can now choose between a walk and a run, each lasting about an hour. You follow a trail of paper, flour, or chalk that has been set ahead of time. There is socializing at the end with food and drink. There is no membership, but a small contribution.

I first heard of the Hash when in Somalia, but I only ran once because I was a slow runner and it was hard to follow the trail in the sand. I was afraid I would get lost. However, I joined Hashes in the other countries where I worked because it was a good way to meet people of all nationalities and a good way to exercise. I even got to know the U.S. Ambassador who ran regularly in the Ugandan Hash.

Exploring Bangladesh

I took advantage of my holidays by exploring some beautiful parts of Bangladesh with my expat friends. We traveled by local train to the northern part of Bangladesh to an area called Sylhet, which had beautiful expansive tea estates. I was always afraid I would miss my train stop due to the language barrier, but we always found someone who spoke English and told us when to get off the train. We had a favorite guesthouse in a British-owned tea estate which had a tennis court, a swimming pool, and lots of places to walk freely. It was a needed rest from Dhaka when it was hot and we needed a respite from the very populated city.

In the southern part of Bangladesh, I toured the mangroves of the Sundarbans with a group of teachers from the international school. We rented a large boat with a cabin where we could all sleep. Our main objective was to see the Royal Bengal tiger. At one point, we got off the boat to walk in the mangrove forest, which was difficult to transverse due to its root system. We hiked to a lookout tower to try and see the tigers. To be honest, I was quite afraid to be off the boat; the local fisherman called them man-eating tigers. Unfortunately, we did not see any, but later another group of expat families saw a tiger, which I heard was a terrifying experience. As I was told, the adults were on the larger boat which was towing a smaller boat with their children. A tiger swam between the big and smaller boat! I am sure it was an unforgettable experience for both the parents and kids.

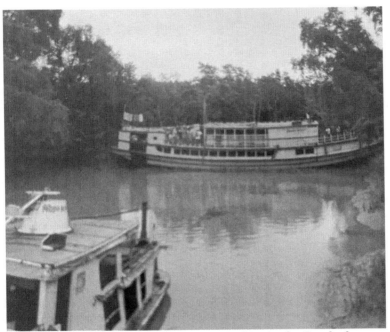

Spent several nights on this boat traveling in the Sundarbans.

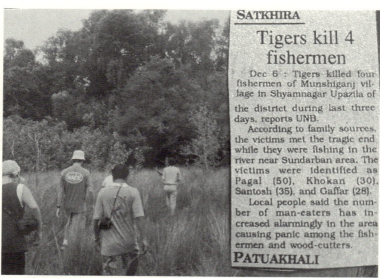

SATKHIRA

Tigers kill 4 fishermen

Dec 6 : Tigers killed four fishermen of Munshiganj village in Shyamnagar Upazila of the district during last three days, reports UNB.

According to family sources, the victims met the tragic end while they were fishing in the river near Sundarban area. The victims were identified as Pagal (50), Khokan (30), Santosh (35), and Gaffar (28).

Local people said the number of man-eaters has increased alarmingly in the area causing panic among the fishermen and wood-cutters.

PATUAKHALI

I hiked to an observation tower looking for Bengal tigers.

Exploring Nearby Countries

India: Bob and I traveled with Alex, Betsy, and some other friends to Calcutta, Darjeeling, and Sikkim in India. In Calcutta, I was shocked and saddened to see men earning money by pulling rickshaws, human-drawn rickshaws not bicycle rickshaws! I went to Mother Teresa's convent in hopes of seeing her, but she was busy at the time. In Darjeeling and Sikkim, we had amazing views of the Himalayas.

Bhutan: On one spring vacation, we traveled to Bhutan where the government organized our travels. It was interesting that the people were not allowed to wear anything but traditional clothes. It was cold then and there was some snow still on the ground. There was no central heating, so we warmed ourselves by the fireplace and were given hot water bottles to take to bed. My favorite memories were watching archery matches, a national sport. The bows and arrows were beautifully made.

An interesting belief in Bhutan was that a wood carved or painted penis represented strength and protection. Wood-carved penises hung from the corners of the roofs of many homes and/or penises were painted on the sides of the homes. You could buy very large wood penises at the market. One was given to me for my birthday!

We toured many monasteries both in Bhutan and Sikkim. I experienced a very different Buddhism than in Thailand. I remember a lot of austere paintings of skulls and pictures that were on the monastery's walls.

Nepal: I went to Nepal several times. One time when I visited with Bob, we rented a plane to fly around Mt. Everest! With my friend Lorrie Byrom and some other friends, we traveled to Nepal and we trekked around Pokhara. We also went to Chitwan Park to ride elephants in order to see rhinos in the wild! The rhinos were not bothered by the elephants so we had a great view of them. After our safari, we got to swim in the river on an elephant bareback.

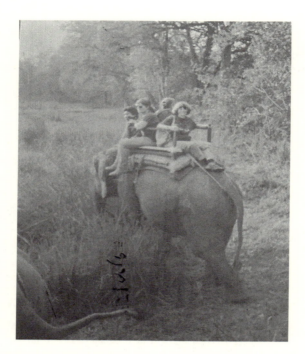

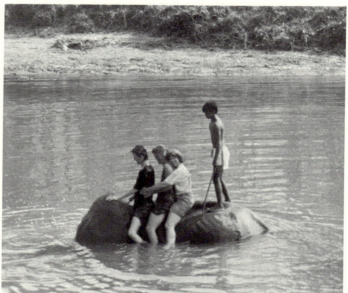

With friends, riding and swimming on elephants in Nepal.

Bali, Indonesia: I visited Bali with Bob and had a wonderful trip. My favorite place was the town of Ubud in the uplands. We got a lovely small cabin perched on a hill with a view of terraced rice paddies and rainforest. I loved visiting the Hindu temples and shrines.

I was sad to leave Bangladesh in October 1995 after four years, but was excited to move on to my next position in Kazakhstan. Bob stayed in Bangladesh until he got a job in Delhi, close enough to Kazakhstan to visit me frequently.

Central Asia Republics - Kazakhstan, Uzbekistan, Kyrgyzstan, Turkmenistan, and Tajikistan December 1995-July 1997

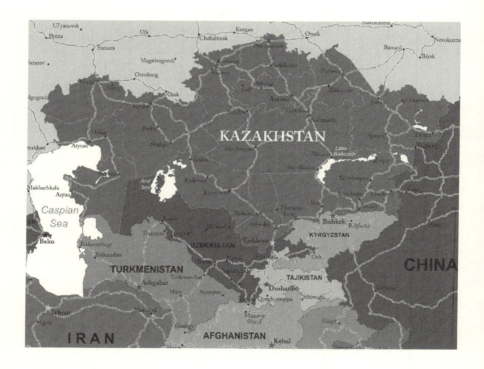

Finding My Next Position and Settling In

Alex, who worked for USAID in Bangladesh, had just been assigned to work in Kazakhstan. He told me about a two-year USAID Personal Service Contractor (PSC) position being advertised as a Reproductive Health Care Program Manager for the Central Asian Republics (CARs): Kazakhstan, Uzbekistan,

Turkmenistan, Kyrgyzstan, and Tajikistan. I would live in Almaty, Kazakhstan where the main office of USAID was located and travel to the other Central Asian Republics. I knew very little about the CARs, but the job description sounded interesting and I met the qualifications for the position. I applied and was accepted. I left Bangladesh in October 1995, spent time in the US, and arrived in Almaty two months later.

The CARs were a part of the Soviet Union until December 26, 1991. I arrived four years after the Soviet Union broke up and the CARs became independent countries. Almaty was still the capital of Kazakhstan. After I left, the capital moved to Astana, now called Nur-Sultan, to be more centrally located in Kazakhstan. I was so fortunate to be able to live in Almaty, it was a stunningly beautiful city! It was surrounded by 13,000- to 16,000-foot snowcapped mountains! The city had many fountains, parks, and tree-lined roads.

I arrived in the middle of a cold and snowy winter and moved into the third floor of a small apartment. The stairwell was dark and dirty and I didn't feel safe until I got into my apartment and locked the door. I was fortunate to have a small screened-in porch that helped make the apartment seem larger and cheerier. A tree was right outside the porch where I hoped to see some birds, however, I rarely saw or heard any. I had a landline, which I was told was probably tapped. I was lucky to have heat which I could regulate. During the Soviet times, the heat was automatically turned off in the spring and turned on in the winter regardless of the weather. If the heat was turned off when it was still cold, the Kazakhstanis would turn on their gas stoves for heat.

For transportation, I didn't own a car, so I walked or hitchhiked. Hitchhiking was the most common form of travel in Almaty. Due to the lack of employment, many local people earned a living by using their own cars as taxis. I felt safe hitchhiking during the day, but was careful at night. I often would be invited to have dinner with Alex and Betsy. As a precaution, when I went home at night, Betsy walked me out to the street and wrote down the taxi's license plate number. She made sure the driver knew she was recording their license plate number.

I had been spoiled by the food in Thailand, Somalia, and Bangladesh and found the food in Kazakhstan not very interesting. I hired a cook who often cooked boiled lamb or beef with a potato dish served with bread. I was told that a meal was not a meal unless you had bread. For picnics, I often ate shashlik (kebabs), which was a stick of beef or mutton cooked over an open fire. On official occasions when Kazakhstanis invited me out for a meal, I was offered horse meat, for there were many wild horses in Kazakhstan, red and/or black caviar, and shots of vodka. I was fortunate enough not to have to eat the eyeball of a sheep, a delicacy offered to honor you! I enjoyed the caviar, which was plentiful and cheap. I had a friend who bought buckets of red and black caviar!

When I first arrived in Kazakhstan, I had to face a new challenge. I started menopause and with it I had a lot of anxiety. I could not concentrate on my work or write reports easily. I had a U.S. Embassy physician who first prescribed anti-anxiety pills, but they didn't help. After one or two months of feeling off, I was prescribed hormone replacement therapy. Thank heaven this worked and I returned to my normal self. This was a great relief.

As I found in Bangladesh, it was easy making friends with other Americans since I worked again in a USAID office. I also made special friends with the staff hired locally which consisted of ethnic Kazakhs, who made up the majority of Kazakhstan's population, and Russians, who were the largest minority in the country. We were both curious and excited to meet each other. They were meeting Americans for the first time and I had never met anyone who was Russian or Kazakh! The local staff were young and well-educated. They spoke Russian, the official language, and English as a second language. I did not speak Russian, as it was not required as a Personal Service Contractor, however, the USAID American foreign service officers were required to speak the language. It did not seem to be a barrier for me because the Kazakhstanis said they loved practicing English with an American. I felt welcomed and embraced. I was pleased when they invited me to join them in their aerobics class after work even though it was taught in Russian. It was fun hitchhiking to the gym together and then trying to follow the instructor's movements!

I made many new friends of all nationalities by again joining the Hash, which had just recently been started. The Kazaks and Russians loved the Hash and outnumbered the expatriates. It was at the Almaty Hash that I was giving my Hash name, Hash Dance, since they all knew I loved to dance. Now when I go to any Hash anywhere in the world, I can announce my name. It is not officially recorded; you just announce it when introducing yourself to the group.

I felt really settled when Alex, Betsy, and my goddaughter moved from Dhaka to living near me in Almaty. I also was very fortunate that my boyfriend, Bob, got a job in New Delhi and was able to visit me frequently. With the arrival of "my family," making new friends at work and at the Hash, my social life was full.

To complete settling in, I decided I needed a pet. I saw many local people walking their dogs. It amazed me that some kept large dogs living in their small apartments, however, walking a dog in the dead of winter was not what I wanted to do. I decided I wanted a kitten. I got prepared and bought food, toys, and kitty litter. I asked a good Russian friend, David, to help me. We looked at ads in the newspaper, made appointments with the owners, and then visited their apartments to see them. I saw mostly Persian cats and was told that their cats were toilet trained (they used toilets rather than litter boxes!). However, I did not feel attracted to any of them. David then took me to an amazing national cat show, but I couldn't get attached to any of them there either. Finally, just before Christmas on a bleak, snowy day, I was with Bob and Betsy at a flea market when we found a Russian blue kitten popping its head out of a cardboard box. I called him Sasha. Many of my Russian friends laughed at the name Sasha, it just was not a common name for a pet.

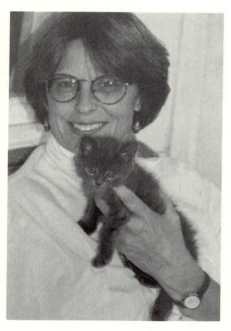

Sasha, a Russian Blue cat, purchased in a flea market in Kazakhstan.

Post-Soviet Era

I learned a lot about the post-Soviet era and the culture of Kazakhstan. It was a hard- financial time for residents and they were desperate for work. There were cadres of people willing to do any kind of work. The U.S. Embassy hired a guard who was an Olympic rowing and sailing coach! Another friend hired a cook who was a surgeon!

Islam was the main religion and the second-most practiced religion was Christianity. Most Christians belonged to the Orthodox Church. During the Soviet times, Christians were not allowed to gather and practice their religion. In August 1995, eight months after I arrived in Almaty, the Kazakhstan constitution was approved, allowing freedom of religion. I was fortunate to be there to attend the FIRST openly celebrated Easter service. There were so many people who wanted to attend that there were not enough seats inside the church. In anticipation for a large crowd, the church set up loudspeakers outside for those who had to stand. I might add it was a cold day. Fortunately, I was able to stand inside the church and watch the service.

Almaty had a stadium called the Hippodrome, where horses were kept, trained, and competed. During Soviet times, the Hippodrome was supported by the Russian government. It was sad to see people struggling to feed and care for the horses. I helped to support the cause by paying for riding lessons. My lessons were in Russian, so I had to learn by imitating the instructor.

I also went with friends to support an international competition held at the Hippodrome. The countries of the CARs were competing in horse jumping, dressage, etc. We dressed up like it was the Kentucky Derby and brought and drank mint juleps. It was a lot of fun watching the horses compete.

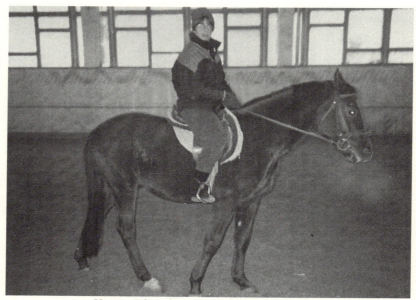

Horse riding lessons in the Hippodrome.

In the Soviet era, the performing arts were well supported. Musicians even had designated buildings with well-equipped rooms in which to practice. In this way they would not disturb their neighbors in their apartment building. They were now old buildings, but were still used. I formed yet another band, the Almighty Cosmic Band, which consisted of expats and local musicians. We rented one of these rooms to practice and was surprised to find a sound system, a drum set, and other equipment available to use. It was interesting to see pictures of bands posted on the wall. There was even a poster of an all-girls band!

In Almaty, the Opera House was still open and offered amazing operas, ballets, and music performances. I spent the equivalent of 50 cents to see a performance, so I went to every single one I could! I saw "Swan Lake" performed with one of the best ballerinas from Moscow. One very interesting performance was an American conducting a Kazakhstani band playing John Philip Sousa marches! The audience had never heard this music before and they loved it. When attending these events, I learned it was custom to check your coat and after the performance you stand in line and wait to retrieve it. I did not do this for the first couple of performances until I noticed I might have been the only one who did not check their coat.

Arasan bath houses for public bathing were very popular. I went frequently in the winter to an old large stone-domed building with Russian, Finnish, and Turkish saunas, with one side of the building for men and one side for women. I joined the local women who were of all ages, shapes, and sizes. You could wear a bathing suit, but most people were naked. I experienced a professional massage by a woman who knelt over me wearing only a bra and underpants and used all her weight as she massaged me. It was too hot for her to wear anything else! On another day, I had a massage on a warm slab of marble; the slabs were heated to different degrees and you could decide which one you preferred. I also experienced using a special sauna where I whipped myself with a branch of oak leaves which was believed to improve circulation and to exfoliate your skin. After the sauna, there was a pool of cold water that you could swim in afterwards. It was so invigorating!

Work Experience

My job was to manage the USAID Project titled "Reproductive Health Service Expansion Project" in the five Central Asian Republics; Kazakhstan, Uzbekistan, Kyrgyzstan, Turkmenistan, and Tajikistan. These five Central Asian Republics are referred to as the "Stans". I did not go to Tajikistan because it was too dangerous due to civil strife among the drug lords.

My responsibility was to oversee an ongoing program to upgrade and expand women's birth control options. The IUD was the most popular contraceptive and abortion was a legal and acceptable form of fertility control. The CARs had a very high literacy rate; their knowledge of contraceptives was limited only because they had been cut off from information from the West. Prior to my arrival, different U.S. organizations had been contracted to implement this project.

I traveled to the different "Stans" and supervised trainings by JHPIEGO, an international NGO affiliated with John's Hopkins, who were responsible to train nurses and doctors how to counsel and provide hormonal contraceptive methods as well as other family planning methods. AVSC trained doctors and nurses on performing female and male sterilization. As the manager of the programs, I observed and assessed the trainings. Since the trainings were mostly conducted in Russian, I needed a translator.

Part of this project was the privatization of pharmacies which promoted the use of the condom. I was not familiar with privatizing pharmacies, but USAID had contracted with an organization called Futures Group International which was implementing the program. My role was reporting their progress based on my observations and their reports.

Shortly after I arrived, the findings of the first Demographic and Health Survey (DHS) in Kazakhstan, Uzbekistan, and Kyrgyzstan were disseminated. This is a nationally representative household survey funded by USAID every five years in countries where they support national reproductive health programs. This survey provided data for a wide range of monitoring, and impact evaluation indicators for population, health, and nutrition. USAID had contracted with a U.S. group called MACRO International, an organization that conducted the DHS in many countries. This was the first baseline survey done in Kazakhstan, Uzbekistan, and Kyrgyzstan. I had never been involved with the writing of a DHS and it gave me the background and experience I needed when I was responsible for overseeing a DHS being conducted in Malawi, which was to be my next position.

I enjoyed traveling to the "Stans." Each country had a resident USAID representative with whom I received a briefing. I observed, assessed, and evaluated program activities. Before I left, I debriefed the country representative with any findings.

I really enjoyed working with the Ministry Health officials in the four republics and coordinating with other international organizations like United Nations Family Population Activities (UNFPA), International Planned Parenthood Federation (IPPF), World Health Organization (WHO), and United Nations Children's Emergency Fund (UNICEF). One of my responsibilities was to ensure the supply of contraceptives in the countries with these organizations.

I did not feel a lot of personal satisfaction working in this position as I had in Thailand, Somalia, and Bangladesh; I discovered I liked the challenge of designing, implementing, and evaluating programs. This position was managing and reporting on an already designed program. More importantly, I was working with an educated population that only needed access to new information, which was done with the use of computers, conducting in-country training, and facilitating doctors and nurses to visit U.S. medical institutions.

Experiences Working and Traveling in the Stans

I felt privileged to work and experience the Stans when they were struggling financially to become independent republics. When I traveled, I stayed in old but functional hotels. It was interesting that there was a "supervisor" sitting on each floor of the hotel watching their customers. I felt like I was being spied on, but maybe they were there to assist. I traveled in national airplanes that were said to not be well maintained such as Kazakh, Uzbek, and Tajik Airlines. In one plane, the seats were not securely fastened so you could turn around and face the row behind you. My friends and I did exactly that, playing cards with friends in the seats behind us! On another plane, the crew had trouble closing an old door before takeoff. On one flight, I was surprised to see a passenger board the plane with a hooded falcon on his shoulder.

I had some memorable times when working in the "Stans." In Uzbekistan, I remember traveling to Samarkand and seeing a beautiful mosque.

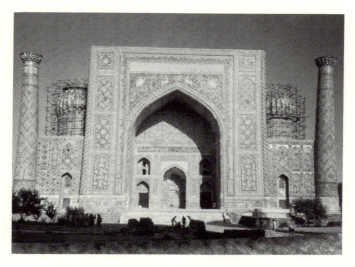

Mosque in Samarkand, Uzbekistan.

In the capital of Turkmenistan, Ashgabat, I remember going to a large outdoor market where camels roamed and amazing handmade rugs and coats were sold.

Traveling in the winter by car to Bishkek, Kyrgyzstan, was a bit scary. We had to cross a snow-swept desolate plain for miles and miles with no one in sight. I was alone with a USAID driver in a four-wheel drive vehicle. We carried blankets and food in case the car broke down enroute. When we arrived in Kyrgyzstan, I felt I had arrived in Switzerland with all the snowcapped mountains. I was amazed that the USAID representative there loved spelunking, exploring the deep caves systems in the mountains using ropes.

In Kazakhstan, one of my more memorable occasions was attending an official dinner with some highly-positioned Kazakh colleagues. We were eating at a long table on an open covered deck overlooking a lake when my colleagues noticed wind and rain coming from an unusual direction. The Hash was cancelled due to this unusual rain. It was suspected that the rain may have been contaminated with radioactivity material. Nine months later, I was shown pictures of some very unusual congenital malformed babies. I informally reported this to local CDC officials, but was told the hospital was a large referral hospital where this was expected. I will always wonder.

Exploring Kazakhstan

My social life was very much integrated with young Kazakhstanis. Alexey, who used to be a former Olympic sail trainer and physical education teacher, loved to take my Kazakh and expatriate colleagues and I rafting, kayaking, sailing, camping, and other outdoor excursions.

Alexey took us rafting down the Ily River in a raft made of two fake rubber torpedoes roped together. As I understand, these fake torpedoes were used during the cold war to confuse the West on the numbers of military equipment that was available.

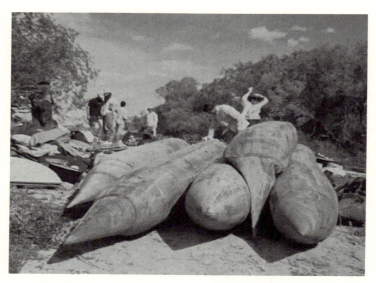

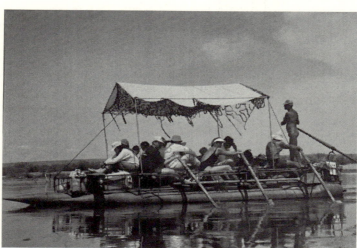

We went down a river on a raft made of fake torpedoes.

We went on an amazing river trip in kayaks that were assembled with wood frames covered with canvas. We saw herds of wild horses on this trip!

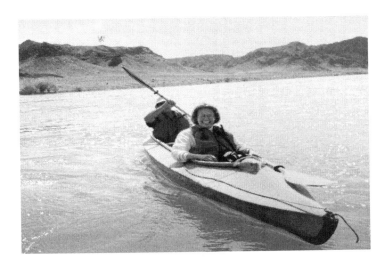

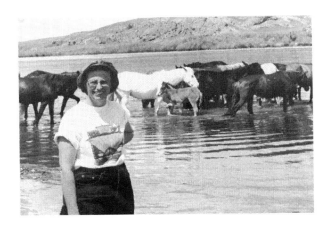

Wood-framed and canvassed-covered kayaks and seeing wild horses.

Our Kazakh and Russian friends organized fabulous trips where we flew in Soviet helicopters, some of the expats questioned the maintenance of the planes, but we were reassured that we had very experienced pilots. One beautiful clear and sunny day, while going for a picnic along a remote river, we flew right over some traditional yurts with men on horseback herding sheep!

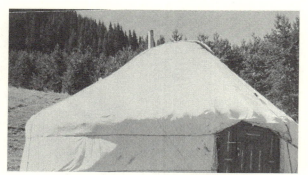

A yurt home seen by helicopter.

One weekend we flew into the Charyn Canyon. I was stunned because it looked just like the Grand Canyon. It was so majestic! We landed and camped along a river where we spent a few nights. Several people drove their Jeeps and brought their kayaks. I wondered how safe it was to kayak because the river looked quite rocky and swift. When I got in the kayak, Alexey told me that someone had rigged a way to catch me before the dangerous section. I only did it once! As we were leaving the canyon and taking our tents down, I was surprised to see scorpions. They had been right under my tent floor!

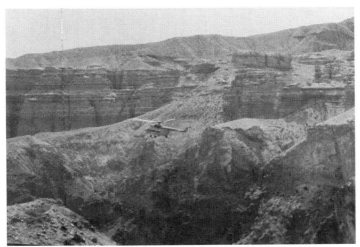

Flying by helicopter into Charyn Canyon.

Alexey also took a group on a sailing trip in a gaff-rigged sailboat on Lake Kapchagay. We sailed for five hours to reach our destination, where we camped for the night. I had a great time in all these trips and am so grateful to Alexey for organizing them!

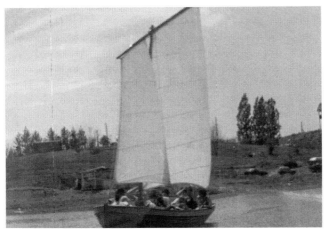

Fun! Five hours sailing in gaff-rigged boat.

During all these excursions, I didn't see much wildlife except wild horses. I was always hoping that I might see a rare snow leopard. Less than 300 were left in Kazakhstan, but I never saw one.

Self-Entertainment

Growing up in rural Vermont prepared me for the outdoor winter adventures. Before I arrived in Kazakhstan, I was advised to bring equipment for downhill and cross-country skiing and skating. I bought new skates and ski equipment and used winter clothes from Goodwill. I was nearing fifty and I hadn't skied much in twenty years! My father had put me on skis as soon as I could walk. I started downhill ski racing in fifth grade and continued through high school and into my first two years at the University of Vermont. Regardless of my skiing history, I was nervous about starting again. We were going to ski at Shymbulak, where the Russian Olympic skiers practiced. Thankfully after my first downhill run, my confidence returned and I was quickly able to ski from the top that involved taking two different chair lifts. The mountain views were breathtaking. On a sunny day, we picnicked at the top, looking at glaciers above and around us. The ski area was not crowded and the expats who skied all knew each other. When we went up on the chair lift, it was fun to cheer the U.S. ambassador learning to snowboard with her son.

There were challenges I didn't expect when skiing. In order to get to the top, we had to take old and rickety single chair lifts with no attendants. I discovered some chairs didn't have seats, so you had to carefully watch and wait for a chair with a seat! Another challenge was driving to and from Shymbulak. It could be very treacherous when the roads were icy because there were few guard rails and the roads were not salted or sanded.

One time I decided to get out of the car and walk, but couldn't even stand on the road without sliding, so I quickly got back into the car and prayed we would get down the hill safely!

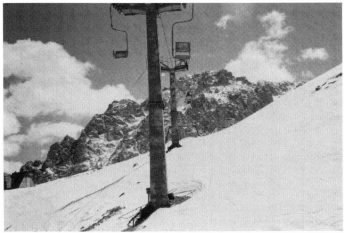

Skiing at Shymbulak.

We skated at Medeu, a famous ice rink used for Olympic training. We cross country skied in apple fields around a dacha that a group of us rented. Dachas were buildings used mostly in the summer by Kazakhstanis to farm and grow their vegetables. They were happy to rent them in the winter. A real plus was that they usually had a sauna!

I was able to continue my love of ballroom dancing. I was fortunate to meet an Arthur Murray instructor who was the U.S. pilot for the president of Kazakhstan. When he was looking for a teaching partner, I volunteered. Each week during my lunch break, he gave me lessons in a huge beautiful empty dance hall in his hotel. On Friday nights, we would then teach dancing at a local bar. We had a loyal following of our Kazakhstani and American friends. It was great fun. My local friend, David, also loved to dance and we even won a prize in a Latin American dance competition!

I celebrated my fiftieth birthday in Kazakhstan. I rented a building in the mountains where the Russian Olympic boxers practiced. The punching bags were taken down so we had a nice large dance hall. I rented a bus so my Kazakhstani friends could come. The Almighty Cosmic Band played and I sang my first solo, "The Loco-Motion" and that night I taught the U.S. Ambassador to line dance! It was a beautiful night and we could see Halley's Comet. Fun was had by all!

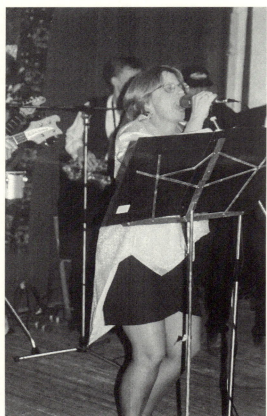

My fiftieth birthday singing in the Almighty Cosmic Band.

Exploring Nearby Countries

I didn't explore the other "Stans" like I did in Kazakhstan, but I did take a memorable trip with friends to Lake Issyk-Kul in Kyrgyzstan in the Tian Shan mountains. During the Soviet time, it was established as a holiday resort for the communist party cadres. This lake is the seventh deepest lake in the world and second largest saline lake after the Caspian Sea. We went out on a cruise boat and I swam in this salty lake. It was very cold and after getting back on board, I was given shots of vodka to warm up! I was told by my Kazakhstani friends that when they learned of this resort, they were shocked at how well the communists had lived before independence. They were told that all people should be equal in their living conditions. It was a real shock to them to learn about their privileged lifestyle.

I traveled to St. Petersburg with Natasha, a young Russian woman who grew up there and now worked at USAID. One day I asked if she would come with me and be my guide and in return I would pay for her flights. She happily agreed! We flew on Aeroflot, which had a bad reputation, but for us it was a luxurious plane compared to Kazakh, Uzbek, and Tajik airlines. I met her family and we toured the major sites. I was blown away by the opulence of the Winter Palace and loved going to see an opera, which thankfully had subtitles for the songs! We both stayed at a hotel because their family apartment was too small to accommodate us. When we left, her family gave me a lovely China teacup and saucer that was their grandmother's. I still treasure this gift, which I still have today. I loved St. Petersburg and it was particularly special having Natasha as my friend and guide. I do regret not exploring Moscow or going to Istanbul, Turkey as many of my friends did.

I left Kazakhstan having great memories. It was hard to say goodbye to all my friends. I was honored by so many gifts from the Kazakhstanis who worked in the USAID office. They came to me one by one to say thank you. I was really touched.

I left Kazakhstan for a position in Malawi. In preparing for my departure, the worst part was getting all the paperwork done to prove my Russian Blue cat was healthy and not a "national treasure." Sasha traveled back with me to Vermont where I saw my father and brother then flew to my home in Olympia, Washington. I was unable to fly with Sasha to Malawi, but later shipped him there by a U.S. Pet transport company. Little did I know Sasha would keep me company for 22 years!

Malawi
July 1997–January 2003

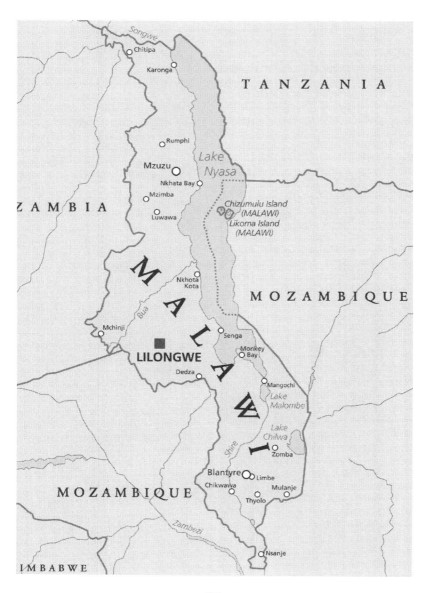

Finding My Next Position and Settling In

I had heard about the position in Malawi from a friend in Kazakhstan. This was now the fourth position I had found out and applied for through word of mouth. This position was as a Senior Reproductive Health Advisor working at USAID in Malawi. It sounded exciting; I would be designing a $26 million reproductive health care and HIV project!

I arrived in Lilongwe, the capital of Malawi, during the winter. I was surprised that it was really chilly in the mornings and evenings. Most houses didn't have any source of heat, but some had a fireplace; however, it became warmer when the sun came up. Bob joined me for the first couple of weeks. It was so much easier emotionally having a partner help me to move into a new country. At first, I stayed in temporary housing, but after a few weeks my supervisor, the USAID health officer, found a perfect small one-story house for me. It had two bedrooms, two bathrooms, a kitchen, and living and dining rooms. The living and dining rooms opened onto a lovely covered patio.

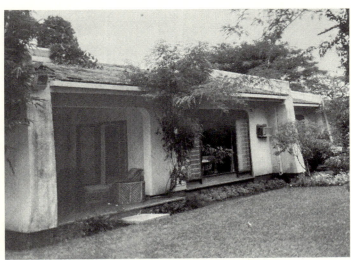

My home in Lilongwe, Malawi.

I had a large yard with lovely yellow flowering acacia trees. I also had a very special cactus called a night-blooming cereus or queen of the night which had grown up a tree like a vine. This was a type of orchid cactus which blooms only at night and wilts the next day; bats are the native pollinators. The cactus has large white flowers--nine inches across! When I thought it was going to bloom, I would invite friends to come over, drink champagne, and sit around the tree to watch it! I loved my cactus! It really made my home special.

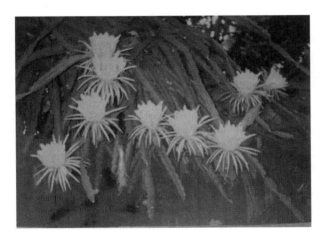

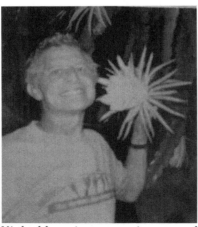

Night-blooming cereus in my yard.

I had all the USAID security measures as I had in Somalia and Bangladesh. Around the house I had a cement wall with barbed-wire on top, security lights, and a twenty-four-hour guard service. All the windows had metal bars and "panic" buttons were installed by my bed, the guest room, and in the living room; if I pushed the buttons, a security team would arrive. I had a special metal door leading to my bedroom that I locked every night before I went to sleep. In addition to these security measures, I had a U.S. Embassy hand-held radio by my bed and a landline phone.

On arrival to Malawi, I bought a reconditioned Toyota Corona. The Japanese send their used cars, usually two years old, to Africa where they are reconditioned and sold cheaply. I later bought a used Land Rover Discovery with high clearance and four-wheel drive necessary for traveling on rough roads. For long trips, I hired a driver who knew the roads and spoke the local language. It broke down several times and got stuck in the mud so I was thankful to have a driver who knew what to do!

As it was in most countries, it was expected you would hire local staff to cook and clean. People were desperate for jobs. When I moved into my house there were already people at my door seeking employment. I was careful when screening staff to try and avoid any chance of theft. I usually hired someone who had worked for an expat and had a good reference. I paid well and treated staff as family. I also hired just one person to have access to the house so that if anything went missing, no one could blame anyone else. However, things happen you never anticipate. I hired a really good cook but when I was away at a conference in Zimbabwe, he took my Toyota Corona, drove it to a bar, picked up some women, and totaled it! Thank heavens no one was hurt. He didn't have a license and luckily, I had car insurance that reimbursed me. The next cook was with me for the remainder of my stay. He and his wife lived in a small house next to mine. He was great!

Shortly after settling in my new home, my cat, Sasha, was flown from Seattle. I had hired a pet transport company to organize his trip and ensure his safe arrival. On his crate was a note that said he had pooped and peed in Amsterdam. I was touched by this extra care. Sasha seemed a bit disoriented, but very glad to see me!

After a few months of living in my new house, Bob decided to quit his job in Delhi and join me. He got a job as a consultant with Population Services International. He was very much in demand and was away for weeks at a time. I made friends through work, participating in the Hash, joining the local sailing club, and learning to play golf at the Lilongwe golf club.

With Bob gone a lot, I decided I wanted the company of a dog. I learned that the South African commissioner had a pregnant beagle and that I should contact him immediately if I was interested in one of the puppies. I contacted him and got the pick of the litter! I named my beagle Snoops.

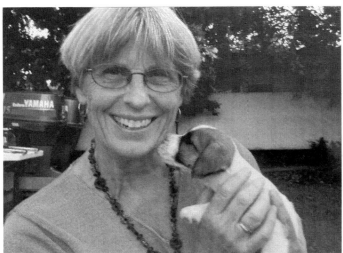

Snoops, my beagle born in Malawi, lived with me for fourteen years.

When I brought Snoops home, I had a puppy shower where people brought toys, newspaper, etc. I was nervous how Sasha would react to Snoops. He first reacted by arching his back and hissing, but in a very short time all was peaceful.

I almost lost Sasha in Malawi. He disappeared for three weeks! My guard told me he often climbed over our gate, which was news to me. We thought maybe Sasha got confused because every house in the neighborhood had a wall around it with a similar gate. Bob and I walked every day in the neighborhood, posted flyers, and put ads on the local radio station. One day a Malawian family found him in their clothes closet! They told me that they had seen him living in the drainage culvert at the entrance of their driveway. They assumed he was a feral cat living on the mice he caught but when Sasha got into their house and hid in their bedroom closet, they knew it must be someone's pet. Their cook remembered one of the radio ads and called my cook. I cannot tell you how happy I was to find him! I gave their cook some reward money.

The USAID office in Lilongwe was an easy drive with little traffic. My supervisor assigned me an office which was my favorite office of all time! It was a large corner office on the third floor with a semi-circular desk, a separate table for meetings and windows along two sides which overlooked the small town. However, there was a disadvantage of having a great view. One day I witnessed "mob justice." I saw many people running after a man yelling "thief! thief!" and then the mob surrounded him and I could no longer see him. I assume they beat him. I learned that "mob justice" was a common way of punishment and there was nothing I could do.

There was another disadvantage of being on the third floor and it was the risk of taking the elevator. One day the USAID Mission Director arrived early in the morning and took the elevator, the electricity went out, and he was stuck for hours. He finally got out when the staff arrived. Ever since, I have tried to avoid taking elevators in countries with unreliable electricity.

HIV/AIDS in Malawi

When I came to Malawi, I experienced the height of the HIV/AIDS pandemic. Unlike in the United States where HIV/AIDS is thought of as a disease among the gay population, in Africa, it is mainly spread by unprotected sex between a man and a woman, transmitted from mother to child through pregnancy, labor, or nursing and spread by blood products through use of unclean needles or unscreened blood.
It is referred to as HIV/AIDs because once you acquire HIV (human immunodeficiency virus) and without treatment, it can progress to AIDs (acquired immunodeficiency syndrome).

At this time in Malawi, there were no free or easily accessible antiretroviral (ARVs) drugs and the number of people who died from the disease was overwhelming. There were so many funerals. Streets were lined with coffin makers. The graveyards were overflowing so some people were considering cremation, even though it was not accepted in the culture. International agencies had to make policies on the number of leave days their local staff could take off to attend funerals. It was difficult for Malawians to follow this policy because they were expected to attend not only their family's funerals, but all their neighbors' funerals too.

A lot of stigma and discrimination was given to those diagnosed with the illness. People feared if their diagnosis was known they would be ostracized, refused treatment and care, or even face abuse and violence. I learned not to ask why someone died because they either did not know or if they suspected HIV/AIDS, it was not discussed.

Work Experience: Support to AIDS and Family Health

I was excited about redesigning a national reproductive health program called "Support to AIDS and Family Health (STAFH)" which had a budget of $26 million to be spent throughout five years. In my first three months, I went on many field trips with the Reproductive Health (RH) Division of the Ministry of Health to assess the current reproductive health program. A formal evaluation of the previous project was also conducted. After this assessment and evaluation, I facilitated a meeting with the RH Division, which prioritized a list of what support they needed to meet their goals and objectives.

I reviewed the RH Division requests with the USAID health officer who helped me determine what was feasible for USAID to support and which USAID funded organizations could provide the necessary technical assistance. I wrote job descriptions for the organizations and approved their key personnel. Once the program was being implemented, my role was to supervise and manage the program to ensure coordination and collaboration with the government. To do this, I facilitated quarterly meetings whereby the selected organizations shared their progress and discussed any issues on implementation with the RH Division. These meetings were extremely useful to help ensure the program was meeting the needs of the government.

One of the most rewarding accomplishments was working with JHPIEGO and the government to improve the infection prevention practices in the hospitals. JHPIEGO was one of the organizations contracted to implement the new amended

STAFH project. JHPIEGO assisted the RH unit to establish national infection prevention standards and a checklist to enable health facilities to do their own assessment of their infection prevention practices. Seven pilot sites were selected at the four central hospitals to pilot the checklist and to assess results.

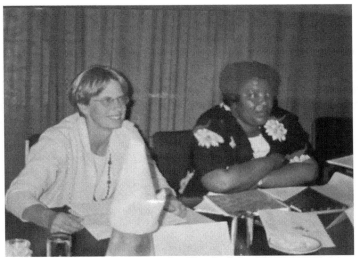

Linda with Jane Namasasu, the Head of the MOH RH Division, at a quarterly coordination meeting.

Using the checklist, one of the hospitals found that used instruments were not being decontaminated prior to cleaning and were not properly being steam sterilized. The instruments were being put into solid metal boxes without any holes which are necessary to allow the steam to enter and sterilize the instruments. JHPIEGO trained the staff to decontaminate instruments prior to cleaning, to clean properly, and purchased sterile drums to replace the metal boxes.

Another hospital identified the need to improve the hospital laundry department. The laundry rooms were disorganized with no system to separate the dirty and clean laundry. The dirty laundry was not decontaminated prior to washing. Those working didn't use proper gloves, gowns, or face masks. It was common to see the sheets drying on the ground around the hospital.

I will always remember the day I visited a laundry department of one of the pilot hospitals. The staff was so happy and proud to show me their gloves, gowns, face masks, and a very clean and organized department. They had dirty laundry coming into one section, a decontamination area, a washing area, and laundry drying on a line. The clean laundry was stored in a separate room with individual shelves marked with the name of the department. The improved morale and pride of the employees in that department was palpable! At the end of this project, all the selected hospitals had greatly improved their infection prevention scores!

Another major accomplishment was working with John Snow, Inc, International (JSI). They had a program called Deliver and had expertise in Reproductive Health Logistics Management and Information systems. JSI hired a Malawian as the Resident Logistic Advisor, who was placed in the Ministry Reproductive Health Unit. He was contracted to improve the logistic management system of contraceptives and drugs to treat sexually transmitted infections (STIs). Depo-Provera was a popular family planning method. It is an injection that has to be given every three months which made it very difficult to keep it properly stocked along with sufficient disposable syringes and needles. I was so pleased when USAID/Washington personnel called and asked me for the reasons the contraceptive prevalence rate seemed to be increasing and I explained I believed it was due to improving the logistic system.

Since there was no accessible treatment for HIV/AIDS, the STAFH project focused on prevention by educating the public and promoting the use of condoms. Condoms were promoted to be used alone or together with other birth control methods. It was critical for the logistics officer to keep the health centers supplied with sufficient condoms as well as the sites outside the health centers such as at truck stops and bars. When I supervised the program, I enjoyed traveling with the logistic advisor to the local bars to stock their supply of condoms. I loved these visits because I had the opportunity to talk with the sex workers and get to know them as people without the label. They also taught me to dance African style!

About a year before I left my position, the USAID Health Office hired a consultant to focus on HIV/AIDS strategies for prevention; the disease was affecting everyone's lives and they really needed a full-time person to manage the program.

My Experience with HIV/AIDS in Malawi

During my six years in Malawi, I learned a lot about the stigma and effects of HIV/AIDS through personal connections. A Malawian colleague had acquired HIV/AIDS and due to stigma, it took a long time before he confided in me that he was HIV positive. I learned he had tested positive a few years back when getting his master's degree in the United States. When he was too sick to work, I visited him at his home and later in the hospital during his last days. As he struggled, he decided he would use his financial resources to secure the expensive antiretroviral drugs, but doing so would deplete the financial resources he would leave for his family. He died before he purchased them. In 2004, one year after I left Malawi, these drugs became free to the public due to the U.S. President's Emergency Plan of AIDS Relief (PEPFAR) under George W. Bush.

When my colleague died, I attended his funeral in his home. I first sat with other women on the floor around his wood casket. I later joined many family members and friends sitting outside the house. People would wail for hours, sharing their grief together. After my colleague's funeral, I went home with a severe headache due to feelings of my own loss and grief.

He left behind a young teenage daughter who I became friends with during her father's illness. After her father died and due to the stigma of HIV/AIDS, I suspected she did not know the real cause of her father's death. I thought a lot about whether or not to discuss this with her. I decided it was important for her to know the truth so she could protect herself. I invited her for a picnic with me in a nearby park. After we had eaten lunch and while we were still sitting on a rock, I gently asked her, "Do you know how your father died?" She said she had been told he died of diarrhea. I explained that her father died of HIV/AIDS, a sexually transmitted disease and explained how it can be prevented. She did not act shocked or surprised. When she went off to boarding school, I wondered how she had accepted what I had told her. One day I was told she had begun an abstinence only group at her school. I feel good that I shared with her how her father died; hopefully, that prevented her and her friends from acquiring HIV/AIDS.

Life Changes

On February 16, 2000 my best friend Pat, who had visited me in Thailand and Somalia, died of ovarian cancer. She was only fifty years old. I had bought a house with her and her friend Carolyn in Olympia, Washington. I wanted a home base when working overseas and this worked out very well for many years. In fact, I bought it sight unseen when I was in Bangladesh. When Pat was diagnosed with cancer, Carolyn kept me updated on her situation. When it looked like Pat was getting very ill, I flew back to help care for her and to give support to her three grown children.

The last trip before she died, I helped organize the music for her service, picked out the urn, found a funeral home for the service, and gathered pictures of her life to display. I was unable to go back for her funeral, but I sent a video of my life in Lilongwe to show at the service. I understand that this brought some laughter. I choose to give a talk on my memories of Pat when sitting on a bench in the Lilongwe National Park. I was unaware that I was near a sign that said "watch out for crocodiles." I ended the video by putting on the golf green on the Lilongwe Golf Course and missed the hole.

When my cook's daughter had a baby, they asked me to name her. I named her Pat. This is a very huge honor in Malawi. Every one of my Malawian friends was impressed that I would be asked to name the baby. Some of my Malawian friend's said I was now Malawian. Through my years working internationally, I was asked to name two more babies. I was visiting a private midwife's clinic in Uganda when I entered into a room with a woman delivering a baby, I was told since I walked in on the delivery, it was custom to ask for the person to name the baby. I named her Rita after my stepmother who died of cancer. In Tanzania, I worked closely with a colleague who asked me to name her baby. I named her Molly, after one of Pat's daughters. I feel so privilege that I got to name three babies after people I loved.

Three months after Pat died, on June 9, 2000, my dad died in Middlebury when I was attending a conference in Nairobi, Kenya. I was staying with friends and before I left, they gave me a tour of the city. When I returned to their house, I found a note that the U.S. Ambassador in Malawi was trying to contact me. I knew something was terribly wrong. I called back to learn my father had died. I first tried to fly back to the U.S. from Nairobi and then Lilongwe, but the flights were full. Even if I could get a flight, I only had a few days of official leave time and it would take two days of flying to get home and another two days to get back, I decided not to go.

However, my brother, Jim, was kind enough to take a video of the service for me. I saw that many of my parent's friends who helped raise me were there and told great stories about my dad. I am still sad that I missed this opportunity to attend the service. To honor him, I asked the administration of the Lilongwe National Park if I could have a small memorial service and plant a tree in his honor. I invited my close Malawian and expat friends to be with me. As we formed a circle around the tree, I shared a brief history of my father and put flowers around the tree. I planted an acacia tree, which would have lovely clusters of small yellow flowers.

I was surprised when I returned months later to see the tree was gone. I learned it had been eaten by a bush pig! I was not upset because my dad, being an outdoorsman, would have laughed.

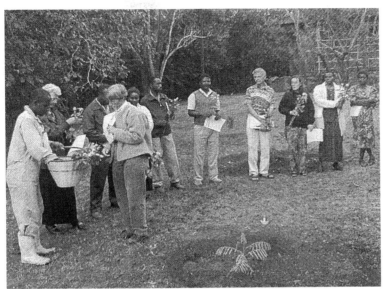

I organized a memorial service for my father and planted a tree in Lilongwe National Park.

The death of Pat and then my father made me anxious and depressed. My anxiety and depression may have been compounded by Larium, a drug I was using for prevention of malaria and was known to have these side effects. The Malawi Peace Corps medical officer told me about one of their volunteers who was a professional counselor. She lived in a rural area outside of Lilongwe. I contacted her and made a deal; I would bring her tuna fish sandwiches in exchange for counseling sessions. She was a lifeline for me. My American neighbors also helped me by recommending I go to their church with them and join the choir. I am so glad I did, because I found singing to be therapeutic. I sang with some wonderful young Malawian women who supported me in my grief and attended my father's service. I also discontinued taking Larium and went back to taking doxycycline. With all this help, I bounced back to normal.

Bob and I split soon after Dad and Pat died. This was also a significant loss after two other losses. We remained friends and later traveled in Spain and France together. After he got married and was living in Tanzania, I found I lived five minutes down the road from their apartment! I was invited for meals on their amazing deck overlooking the ocean and ate out at their favorite Indian and Japanese restaurants. When I retired and was diagnosed with cancer, Bob came to visit me. I am so grateful we have remained friends.

After Bob left and we both had moved on in our lives, I started dating Ziggy, whom I met at the Hash. He was from Zimbabwe where his family owned a commercial farm. He was trained in Europe to repair computers and came to Lilongwe where he started his own computer store. He was a single father supporting his two teenage daughters.

Living Overseas Had its Own Risks

Attempted Robberies

Only in Malawi was my security breached and it was breached twice. One night while I was sleeping, someone pried open the bars on the living room window and reached in and stole my music system, which was in front of the window. I was glad I was securely locked in my bedroom in case they had entered the house. I learned not to place anything valuable near the window. It was a creepy feeling to know they climbed my fence or gate and were able to get into my yard while I was sleeping!

I also had an attempted robbery by a gang of thieves which was very traumatic. It was in the early evening when I was home alone. I hadn't locked the front door because Snoops, my beagle, was still coming in and out of the house. I was in the living room talking on the phone to Ziggy. As I was talking, I heard someone at the door and looked up to see six or more men dressed as policemen at my front door. Before I could stand, they rushed in and came running toward me. I screamed! Someone pulled the phone cord out of the wall and tied my hands behind me. Someone else held me down on the floor with their hands around my neck. They asked me where the keys of the car were and where I kept my money and alcohol. The men took my valuables and put them in my Land Rover. While I was being held on the floor, I prayed they wouldn't rape me and that Ziggy heard my scream and would come. I was so relieved when I heard a truck screeching around the nearby corner. The men heard it too and ran out of the house. Then there was silence. I later understood that the guard would not let Ziggy into my compound until all the men were hidden behind the guardhouse near the gate. Meanwhile Ziggy climbed on the roof of his truck and asked the guard, "What is going on?" When the guard opened the gate, the men all ran out of the compound. Ziggy ran after them with his gun.

Ziggy had brought his teenage daughter with him, who came into the house and found me on the floor with my hands tied. When I was untied, I called Sheila, a close friend who was the medical officer for the Peace Corps in Malawi. She came immediately. She pushed the "panic" button and a security team came to the house. Since the thieves ran away, I didn't lose my Land Rover and all the things they had put in it and I was so thankful they did not rape me which was my biggest fear. Whether my guard was involved in the heist or forced to allow the robbers in, I do not know, but he was put in jail for accessory to the robbery.

After they left, I couldn't find Sasha and panicked, but later found him hidden under my bed in a space between the mattress and springs. It took me some time to coax him out.

Snoops seemed fine. I was in shock. I couldn't eat and could only drink from a straw due to the trauma to my neck. The USAID health unit flew in an American psychiatrist from South Africa to counsel me. After a few visits, I found a Canadian counselor in Lilongwe and continued my counseling. I had a South African friend named Rusty, who came and stayed with me at the house until I felt safe to be alone again. Sheila was always checking up on me, too.

The thieves were caught after robbing another house in the area where an occupant recognized one of the robbers. She kept her head down and after the robbers left, she reported him. The police caught him and he named the others. After I knew they were all in jail, I finally felt safe to live in my house. I also felt safe walking in town knowing they were not watching me. After this incident, the USAID security team further strengthened my security by cutting down some limbs of the trees that might help robbers to climb over my wall.

Personal Experiences with Tropical Diseases

One of the most amazing people I met in Malawi was Sheila, who provided me with support during and after the robbery. She was a British nurse who was trained and qualified as a physician assistant in the U.S. She worked for many years in Malawi and other countries as the medical officer for Peace Corps. She was an amazing clinician and saved many lives. I learned a lot from her about the following tropical diseases which I had never had any experiences with before Malawi.

Bilharzia/Schistosomiasis

I swam frequently in Lake Malawi, also known as Lake Nyasa, where bilharzia, also called schistosomiasis, was very prevalent. This is a serious disease caused by parasites that are carried by freshwater snails. When they come in contact with your skin, they enter your blood vessels and can then travel to many parts of your body causing many different symptoms. They can even travel to your brain and spine causing seizures and paralysis. Sheila recommended that I take prophylactic medicine every six months which I did!

I didn't contract bilharzia in Malawi when taking prophylactic medicine. However, when I moved to Uganda, I swam in Lake Victoria where I contracted a mild case and was treated. I decided to stop swimming and sailing in Lake Victoria because I didn't want to restart taking preventative medicine every six months.

Malaria

When I arrived in Malawi, I started taking doxycycline to prevent contracting malaria. I took it every day for almost ten years except when I tried Larium, which I quit because of the side effects. Malaria can be a fatal disease caused by the anopheles' mosquito. Since these mosquitoes are known to be more active in the evening, night, and early morning, I applied mosquito repellent every evening before going outside and slept under a mosquito net. I also had screens on my windows and my housekeeper frequently sprayed the house with insecticide. I took medication while working in Malawi and later in Uganda, but I quit when I went to Tanzania; I decided I had been on doxycycline too long. However, I always adhered to using repellent when outside in the evenings and slept under a net. I was very fortunate to avoid getting malaria while living in Africa. However, I did recommend to my family and friends who visited for a short time to take medication to help prevent malaria. Why ruin a vacation?

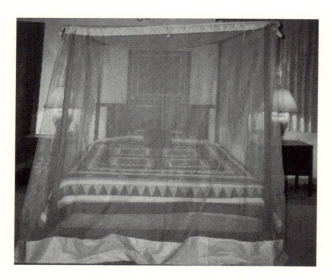

Mosquito net over my bed.

Rabies

Sheila recommended I get the rabies vaccine because many dogs in developing countries are not vaccinated against the disease. If bitten and not treated immediately, rabies is usually fatal. I will never forget one incident that happened in Malawi. While visiting a very rural health clinic, I met a father who was frantic because his son had been bitten by a rabid dog. He said the dog had just come running around their outhouse and attacked his son. He had just learned there was no treatment at this center, but there was treatment in a larger hospital in the next town. Since the father and son had no transportation, I offered to take them there. When we arrived, we were informed that the rabies shots were very expensive. The father told me he would sell some of his land so his son could have the necessary injections. I knew the family was poor and this was a huge sacrifice, so I paid for it. The father was so grateful and I felt good I was able to contribute. This was my one and only encounter with a rabid dog, thank heavens!

Personal Experiences with African Wildlife

For the first time, I not only had personal experiences with tropical diseases, but I had close encounters with some of the wildlife which I loved and respected.

Close Encounters with Hippopotamuses

Lake Malawi was the focus of my outdoor activity, but there were associated risks when in the water. Besides the risk of contracting bilharzia, there were hippos and crocodiles. Sheila had access to a cottage on Lake Malawi where I spent many weekends. There was a resident hippo that would swim up and down the beach at certain times of the day and we would have to time our swimming in order to avoid him. Prior to my time in Malawi, up the beach from Sheila's, some kids were playing with innertubes, one dove down and never came up. This drowning was thought to be due to a hippo.

Unknowingly, I almost waterskied over a hippo when I was having a birthday party at the lake! I was asked if I wanted to waterski; I had not waterskied for years. I got up on two skis with no problems, kicked a ski off, and slalomed back and forth over the wake of the boat. I was so pleased with myself! When I landed on the beach, I was hoping my friends would be impressed, but instead I was greeted with, "you just missed skiing over the hippo! Didn't you see it?" I had never thought of looking for hippos while waterskiing!

Ziggy was the commodore and I was the vice commodore of the sailing club on the Lilongwe Water Reservoir. It was very popular among families; the kids learned to sail and practiced capsizing and rescues. The club lost popularity when some of the kids contracted bilharzia and could no longer swim in the water. The enthusiasm also waned for sailing due to a single male (bull) hippo who took up residency. Some members still sailed, but would have someone on shore to track the hippo with binoculars. If the hippo started to follow the boats, the sailors were signaled to come into shore.

Ziggy and I loved the club and continued to sail despite the risks. One day he invited me to sail in his catamaran up the inlet of the reservoir. While we were sailing, I asked Ziggy, "Have you seen the hippo?" All of a sudden, the sailboat lurched and we realized we had just sailed over it! That was the last day I sailed at the dam!

Close Encounters with Crocodiles

One day a very large crocodile was found sunning itself on the lawn of the sailing club. Ziggy had brought his gun and gave a warning shot. The croc leaped into the air and left, but we had no idea where it went! It was now very hard to get anyone to come and join the sailing club with the water contaminated with bilharzia, a resident bull hippo, and now a large crocodile.

I often rented a cottage on Lake Malawi called the Wheel House, which kept a resident crocodile in a pool. On my birthday, I rented this cottage and invited my friends. When I arrived, I learned that the crocodile had escaped a few weeks earlier and the owners didn't know where it had gone. They thought it had moved to the southern part of the lake. As part of the birthday festivities, I rented local dugout canoes for a race. Little did I know how difficult it was to keep these canoes upright and to paddle. It was a bit scary knowing the croc might be around! Thankfully we all had fun and were safe.

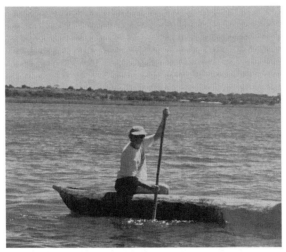

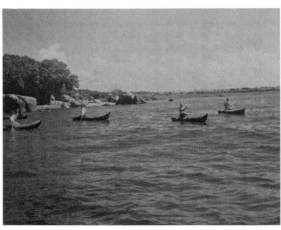

Dugout canoe race on Lake Malawi.

I learned from a taxi driver in Seattle that Lake Malawi was famous for its tropical fish. They were harvested in the lake and sold throughout the world. I learned where they harvested the fish. I went out by boat with friends and spent hours snorkeling and looking at these beautiful fish. I didn't know until later that there was a high risk of crocodiles in the area. Ziggy told me he stayed on the boat in order to watch for them. Yikes! I am so lucky I didn't encounter a crocodile!

Experiences with Elephants

I went on many safaris in Malawi and southern Zambia where I became respectful of elephants. During my time in Malawi, a young local safari guide, known by many friends, was killed by an elephant. He was taking a group on a walking safari and instructed the group to walk close behind him, but one of the tourists walked away to take pictures. An elephant charged him. The guide ran between the elephant and tourist and shot his gun in the air which would normally scare the elephant away, but this time the elephant charged and killed the guide. Many of my friends knew the guide and mourned his loss.

On one safari in Malawi, I observed that the driver kept a good distance from the elephants. He stopped the Jeep where he could get a quick getaway and I asked him why. He told me there was an elephant called Mary, who was very aggressive and would charge vehicles. He said elephants in the area were aggressive because they had been injured or maltreated by farmers who wanted to chase them away from eating or destroying their crops. During that same safari, we got stuck in the mud in the middle of the park when it was getting dark. I was really scared!

After these experiences, I requested the safari guides to not drive too close to the elephants or other wildlife. If it was a walking safari, I walked right behind the guide. Even though I have fears around elephants, I still love and admire them. They are amazing intelligent creatures with some of the same emotions as humans. Through the years, sadly I have seen the number of elephants dwindling due to poachers. I now wear a t-shirt that says "Only elephants should wear ivory."

Experiences with Snakes and Spiders

Snakes were not often seen in the city because they were immediately killed whether or not they were venomous. However, one day when I was with Ziggy, his daughter called and reported a Mozambique spitting cobra on a friend's deck. Ziggy immediately called the local snake expert who came and confirmed it was a spitting cobra. He captured it, and released it in a safe place. My brother, Jim, being a herpetologist met this expert and learned about the snakes in Malawi. Jim later encountered a snake when bathing in an outdoor shower. It took him by surprise, but thankfully, he learned it was harmless.

I only saw two very large hairy spiders in the twenty-eight years working overseas and I was lucky because I am deathly afraid of them. One evening when living in Bangladesh, I looked up and saw one on my ceiling; I tried to hit it with a broom, but it escaped. I had to sleep through the night wondering where it was. In the morning it was coming up the stairs to my bedroom, I killed it with my tennis racket.

The second one I saw in my home in Malawi. I was working at the dining room table with the doors open to the patio. Snoops started barking. I said, "Snoops be quiet!" He kept barking. I looked up from my computer and there on the floor next to me was a huge spider. I am sorry to say we killed it.

Self-Entertaining

I hosted many parties with my Malawian colleagues, but my Christmas parties were the most popular. I introduced the "Yankee Swap," where everyone brought a wrapped present under $5 and placed it under my fake Christmas tree. Each person was given a number and when their number was called, they would either take a gift under the tree or take someone else's gift. One year, I wrapped a live chicken in a box with holes and another year I wrapped a gift card for a goat, which I hid outside. It was so much fun! Every year the Yankee swap became more and more popular!

As I did in Bangladesh, I found a Mother Teresa orphanage and three or four times a year gathered expat friends to visit and play with the children. One time, I brought them to my house for an American-style picnic and served hamburgers. This was a great success! Prior to Christmas, we provided money for a special chicken dinner, and early Christmas morning we brought presents for the children. It was a special way to celebrate the holiday!

When I arrived, Bob and I became good friends with the U.S. Ambassador's secretary and then became friends with the Ambassador herself. On July 4, the Ambassador would invite all the Peace Corps volunteers for a picnic at her house. One year she asked me to teach the volunteers line dancing on the tennis court! That was a hoot! Bob and I often were invited to the Ambassador's house for dinner and game nights which were really fun. We helped to decorate her residence for the Christmas holidays and participated in her annual caroling. She didn't play tennis, but she generously allowed others to enjoy her tennis courts. I often played tennis while listening to local African drumming in the nearby villages. I loved it and felt so fortunate!

I learned to play golf at the Lilongwe Golf Club, where I took lessons from a Malawian golf instructor. He was an excellent teacher, however, he had a drinking problem, so I took lessons in the morning when he was sober. I became hooked playing golf and continued to play golf for the rest of my time in Africa; you can play 360 days a year! I did have one unfortunate accident when playing golf in Malawi. When I took my tee shot, I killed a bird with my golf ball! I was very upset and to make matters worse, I watched a bird of prey swoop down and fly off with it.

Bob and I did some kayaking with friends on Lake Malawi. We traveled with them to some beautiful pristine islands located within the Lake Malawi National Park. This area was set aside for the protection of freshwater fish. We stayed at Mumbo Island camp which partnered with Malawi's Department of National Parks and Wildlife. They had lovely tents, no electricity, and had eco-friendly compost toilets. We all went snorkeling; the water was crystal clear and it was reported that there was no bilharzia in this part of the lake.

Exploring Outside Malawi

Zimbabwe

On Bob's fiftieth birthday, we flew to Harare, stayed at the famous Meikles Hotel and then flew to Victoria Falls where we stayed at the famous old colonial Victoria Falls Hotel. It was a grand hotel where I experienced traditional high tea with scones, whipped butter, cakes, and tea! Yum! We had many adventures there. We walked to the Falls trying to avoid the baboons, which were large and I didn't trust. We watched bungee jumping which was frightening even to watch and we had a scary adventure ourselves. We decided to go canoeing on the Zambezi River above the Falls. There were not enough guides for the canoes, so because I was an experienced canoeist, they asked me to paddle with Bob. We were warned there were many pods of hippos we must avoid. We then took off down the river. We were to stop at an island, but left due to a large bull elephant on the shore with ears flapping. As we continued downstream, I became aware that the sound of the Falls was getting louder and louder. I asked, "When are we going to pull out of the river?" but I had no response. Between worrying about the hippos, the elephant, and now the Falls approaching, I was a nervous wreck. Why did I decide to do this?! We got out safely, but I wondered what was I thinking?

However, Bob and I later decided to take a helicopter ride to see the Falls from the air. What I did not realize is that the river was very shallow at the top of the Falls and you could walk above them on the rocks. I wish I had known this before our canoe trip! We also took a peaceful sunset cruise on the Zambezi River. Now that was a very relaxing trip!

South Africa

I traveled to South Africa frequently. There were conferences I attended in Pretoria and Cape Town. In Pretoria, the crime rate was very high. My friends, whom I stayed with, had extremely tight security in their homes. Cape Town felt safe to me. One conference I attended was in winter and it snowed! There was no heating in the hotel and it was so cold. I also went to Cape Town as a tourist. I visited Robbin's Island, took the gondola up to the top of Table Mountain, traveled along the coast to see Jack Ass penguins, and enjoyed the wine country!

I visited Johannesburg (Joburg) for medical care. I tore my meniscus and went there for knee surgery. I was fortunate to be able to stay with the U.S. Embassy health unit doctor who I had known from my Bangladesh days. They looked after me in the hospital and I stayed with them until I could fly home.

There were only a few stores in Lilongwe, so it was also fun to fly to Joburg at Christmas time to shop. Sheila would buy hams for Christmas dinner and presents for her daughter and she invited me along on one of these trips. I was surprised to find the flight was full of people I knew all going to Joburg to prepare for the holiday. It was a great time!

One year, Ziggy and I also drove to Joburg at Christmas time to buy presents for his daughters. It was quite an adventure; we had to carry our own fuel for one section of the trip. We stopped first to see his relatives in Harare then went on to Joburg. After Joburg we went out to the coast to see if we could see the sea turtles lay eggs and then drove to and explored Durban. We came back visiting some nice remote beaches in Mozambique. I loved this adventure!

Zambia

South Luangwa National Game Park in Zambia was my favorite park for wildlife. It is off the beaten track with few tourists and they had personalized safari trips. Bob and I drove their many times. We took my brother, Jim, and his wife, Kris, there when they came to visit me in Malawi. We stayed in a camp within the park along a river. Hippos would come out of the water to graze at night. They were the most dangerous on land for they would charge you if you came between them and the river. If you wanted to travel from your cabin to the main lodge, you needed a guard escort.

I again had an elephant scare. On one of our drives in the park, a young elephant came out of the bush and chased us. Our driver wanted to teach this young elephant to not chase vehicles, so he would start and stop the Jeep until the elephant just stopped chasing us. I was not very happy with this elephant training.

I always wanted to see wild dogs. One night I decided to not go on the night safari. Aunt Ellen, my mother's sister, had recently died and I wanted time alone to write a condolence letter to my cousins. It was that night Kris, Jim, and Bob saw wild dogs! I was green with envy! They are very rare to see. While they were seeing wild dogs, I was alone in my cabin when I heard the loud roar of lions. It sounded like they were right outside my cabin. I didn't know what to do, so I locked myself in the bathroom, scared to death. Later I learned they were not so near my cabin, but I can say I have heard roaring lions in the wild!

Leaving Malawi

I worked for five years with USAID, which is the time limit set for Personal Service Contactors. However, I didn't want to leave my friends and colleagues! I wanted to settle down and retire there. I stayed for an extra year and tried to start an NGO. Malawi had a high maternal mortality rate and one reason was a critical shortage of nurses/midwives who had left the hospitals due to the poor government working conditions. The goal of the NGO was to bring nurses back into the profession, train them to ensure quality of care, and assist

122

them to start their own private practice. This was being done successfully in Uganda.

Since I was no longer working for USAID, I had to move out of my house. I found a friend who offered to share his house with me. I worked in partnership with the Malawi Nursing Council and Nursing schools. We formed an amazing board, wrote a constitution, and applied for NGO status. However, the timing wasn't right; the Malawi government had decided to limit the number of local NGOs and we needed that status to receive international funding. I no longer could afford to work without a salary and decided to seek other work.

Uganda
February 2003–September 2006

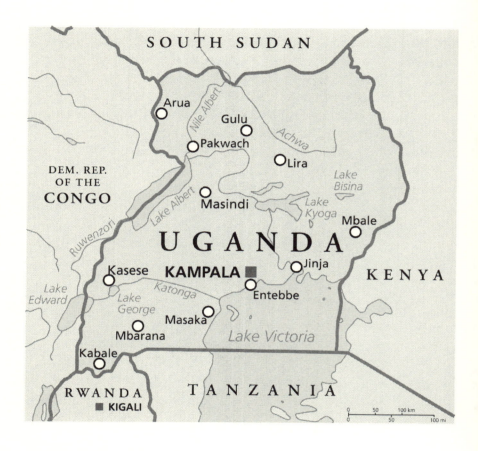

Finding My Next Position and Settling In

I found and applied for my next job online. Right after I had sent in my application, I was called for a phone interview! The position was for a Senior Technical Advisor to the Elizabeth Glaser Pediatric AIDS Foundation (EGPAF) in Uganda and was funded by the Population Leadership Program. The job was to integrate family planning into the national Prevention of Mother to Child Transmission (PMTCT) of HIV Program. It sounded like a perfect fit for me! They offered me the position and I accepted.

However, in accepting this position, I knew I would have to part ways with Ziggy and his family. He wanted to pursue his dream to have a farm. He ended up buying a farm in George, South Africa, a lovely town along the coast called the Garden Route. I visited him once when I was living in Uganda and he gave me a tour of the famous Garden Route and his farm. We are still friends on Facebook.

I arrived with Snoops and Sasha in Kampala, Uganda's capital. The morning after I arrived, I was greeted by my friend Rob, who I had worked with in Bangladesh, and who was now the Health Officer for USAID in Uganda! Rob picked me up at the hotel, took me out for breakfast, and showed me around the city. It was a great way to start a new position!

With a local realtor, I found a beautiful modern wood home in a compound with another similar house, both were designed and owned by a Swiss architect. It had the standard security measures, a secure wall around the compound with security lights, barred windows, panic buttons and a twenty-four-hour guard. I also now had my first cellphone, which gave me a real sense of security!

The most attractive part of the house was a large porch that overlooked a big, sloping yard. The yard was big enough to set up two badminton courts for parties, one court for kids and one for adults. There were lovely trees in the yard. My favorite tree was the tulip tree, producing red tulip-shaped flowers about two inches in diameter. It bloomed in May and June, so this is when I knew it was spring.

I was very fortunate that the house next door was occupied by a wonderful American family with their two young sons. They included me as part of their family by sharing morning coffee, co-hosting badminton parties, and celebrating holidays. Snoops had lots of attention and loved running between houses.

I hired a wonderful woman who cleaned and cooked for me. I wanted to keep the Land Rover I had purchased in Malawi, so I hired a driver to drive it to Kampala. I also hired a full-time driver to take me to work each morning because of the heavy traffic which enabled me to start my day's work in the car. He also drove me on many field trips.

When I started my position, the EGPAF office was downtown, located in a new modern multi-story high rise office building. EGPAF had rented a small space with a fabulous view on the fourteenth floor. I must mention that I climbed the stairs every day out of fear of a power outage and being stuck in the elevator, however, when I sprained my ankle and had to use crutches, there was no choice but to use it. I shared a room with two physicians, one from Uganda and one from Rwanda, both of whom provided me with lots of support and advice.

Our office staff grew as more employees were hired for new projects, so we moved to a converted one-story house away from downtown Kampala. I was happy because there was no elevator! Our country director was a very experienced, kind, and thoughtful British man. I now shared a room with a Ugandan obstetrician and a Ugandan pediatrician. The pediatrician impressed me. He was young, handsome and had recently received his master's in public health from Berkley. He loved camping in the bush and taking photographs of the wildlife!

Work experience

I worked for almost four years with the Elizabeth Glaser Pediatric AIDS Foundation. I loved the challenge of designing and implementing a new national program to integrate family planning (FP) into the Prevention of Mother to Child Transmission (PMTCT) of HIV Program.

I used all the lessons I had learned in the other countries; identify and meet the key government officials and NGOs involved in FP and PMTCT, assess the government's level of interest and commitment, listen and learn from the experts in the field, and develop a team to implement and evaluate the program. I first made an appointment with the head of Reproductive Health Division of the Ministry of Health. We introduced ourselves; I learned he was a physician with his master's in public health from Tulane University. (I mention his educational background because I am always humbled by the fact that many of the people I worked with have more education and experience than I do.) I explained that I was working for EGPAF and had received $250,000 that could be spent for integrating family planning services into their PMTCT program. I asked him if he thought this was a program that was needed in Uganda. I think he was surprised and pleased to be asked. He agreed this was very much needed and encouraged me to talk with the physician in charge of PMTCT in the government's AIDS Control Program. From that day on, he always fit me into his busy schedule when I needed his advice; this meant to me that he was committed to the program.

The next day I made an appointment with the program officer of the PMTCT program. When I met her, she said, "Why not fly with me tomorrow to the northeastern part of Uganda to observe a PMTCT training?" I felt so fortunate to have just arrived in Uganda and to be immediately invited to fly with her for a site visit. This was amazing!

Background of the PMTCT Program

In Uganda, mother to child transmission of HIV was a major health problem. HIV can be transmitted from a HIV positive mother to a child during pregnancy, childbirth, or breast feeding. According to the Uganda Bureau of Statistics 2000/2001, the total estimated population was 24.7 million people and approximately 1.3 million adult females would get pregnant every year. With a prevalence of HIV of 6.2 percent (Uganda HIV Sentinel Surveillance Report 2002) it was expected there would be 85,000 HIV positive pregnant women every year and 30 percent of these women would pass on the infection to their babies if there were no interventions. This would be an estimated 25,000 HIV positive babies would be born each year with no interventions. Two thirds of those babies will be dead by their second birthday. [4]

The Prevention of Mother to Child Transmission (PMTCT) of HIV was a relatively new program; it was rolled out in the year 2000, or three years before I arrived in Uganda. A new drug had been developed called Nevirapine, which if taken as a single dose by the HIV positive mother at the onset of labor and given to the baby after delivery was shown to reduce the risk of HIV transmission from mother to child by almost 50 percent. However, this resulted in more babies born with no one to care

[4] Ministry of Health, Strengthening Family Planning within The PMTCT Program in Uganda, Trainee Handbook July 25, 2005, pg 6

for them. Without treatment, Antiretroviral drugs, many HIV positive mothers died and the grandmothers, who were expected to care for the babies if the mother died, didn't have the resources or were not healthy enough to care them. The number of orphanages was growing. However, this all changed one year after I arrived. In 2004, due to the U.S. President's Emergency Plan of AIDS Relief (PEPFAR) under President George W. Bush, free antiretroviral (ARV) drugs became available for adults and the mothers could be treated and kept alive to care for their children.

I had a very personal experience on the introduction and impact of the free ARVs. In May 2004, during the PMTCT international video conference, which I will discuss later, a woman stood up and disclosed she was a HIV positive mother and that she wanted to live to see her children grow up, but could not afford to buy ARVs. Her story so touched me that right after the conference, I wrote and gave her a note offering to pay for her treatment. I then had to research where she could get the drugs and the cost. We eventually agreed on a provider and she started her ARVs. I supported her for several months and then one day she called me and told me she had found a place that was offering free ARVs. We were both excited! I kept in touch with her and later learned that her husband was HIV negative, they were what we called a discordant couple. She and her husband went on to become well known, outspoken public figures providing support to other HIV positive women and discordant couples. I was so proud of her and her husband. It was great news to learn free ARVs were becoming available!

Integrating Family Planning into PMTC

Preventing unintended pregnancies among HIV positive women was an important strategy to prevent mother to child transmission. The contraceptive prevalence rate in Uganda was very low; 23 percent of currently married women were using some form of contraception but only 18 percent were using a modern method. (Uganda DHS 2001)

A USAID funded analysis that had been done during this time examined the costs and benefits of adding family planning services to PMTCT. The findings suggest that the addition could save lives of thousands of women and children and significantly reduce the number of orphans. It was one of the World Health Organizations global strategies to prevent PMTCT.

Observing the PMTCT Training Program at Soroti Regional Hospital

The doctor in charge of the PMTCT program and I flew to Soroti Regional Hospital. We sat together on the plane and this gave us both an opportunity to get to know each other.

I learned a lot about PMTCT on this visit, both in the classroom and in the prenatal clinics. (In Uganda and in many countries, prenatal is commonly referred to as antenatal.) One of the key researchers for Nevirapine was a well renowned and respected Ugandan pediatrician, who taught the PMTCT class. I was getting the latest and most up to date information. I observed the counseling in the prenatal clinics where women were being tested for HIV/AIDS and listened to women being told for the first time they were HIV positive. They were devastated. They would say, "I cannot tell my husband; he will leave me. Who will help me raise the children?"

I realized it was not an appropriate time to bring up family planning with prenatal women when they were dealing with their new diagnosis. At every meal break, I would brainstorm ways to integrate family planning with the head of the PMTCT program and others, but no one could come up with a plan. I felt stuck!

As a result of this visit, the head of the PMTCT program and I became good friends. We bonded over an incident which we laughed about through the years that we worked together. This occurred after the first night of training when she asked me, "How was it taking a bath? "I admitted it did not go well. I explained that I took the bucket of warm water which was brought to me, filled the large plastic bowl that was in the bathroom, and poured the whole bowl over my head. I got all the towels and everything wet! She laughed and informed me that you cup your hands to scoop the water up from the bucket to wash yourself. I tried this method, but just could not do it. She then found a cup for me to use. I made sure that on my future field trips, I always carried a cup!

Learning From Other African Countries

Fortunately, I heard of an international non-profit organization in Cape Town, South Africa, called "mothers2mothers," a program where they trained HIV positive mothers as mentors for other HIV positive mothers. They had developed a training curriculum for mentors which included family planning. The mentors worked as community health workers and they led support groups. I decided I had to go to Cape Town to study and observe this program. I went and talked to many of the woman about their thoughts and feelings regarding peer support. The feedback was overwhelmingly positive and they discussed and used family planning. After my return to Uganda, I heard about three other small scale NGOS in Cameroon, Zimbabwe, and Tanzania, who had started peer support groups for pregnant HIV positive mothers.

I decided the best way for the four NGOs in four different countries to share lessons learned and insights with Ugandan government officials and Ugandan NGOs was to organize an international video conference. Each invited NGO would present a slideshow of their peer support group and how they addressed family planning. The biggest obstacle was the logistics; each organization in each country had to find and to travel to a video conference center which had the appropriate technology and personnel to use that technology.

Fortunately, in Uganda, near the EGPAF office, WHO had a large auditorium with a wall-size screen. There was a well-trained technician who could help connect the four countries. All the NGOs in Kampala, who were involved in addressing HIV/AIDS and PMTCT, were invited. On the day of the conference, I was so happy to see the auditorium was packed! Government officials from the Reproductive Health Division and AIDS Control Program led the meeting. We all learned how peer support groups assisted women/couples to accept their diagnosis, decreased depression, reduced stigma and discrimination, increased disclosure to their husbands, family, and friends, and discussed and encouraged family planning. We also learned how this helps the pregnant women to better manage those conditions that will affect her pregnancy and to provide an easy way for health providers to follow up women/couples and their families. It was pointed out that support groups were cost effective because they use a minimum of resources. At the end of the conference, the physician in charge of the PMTCT program and the Reproductive Health Division requested that EGPAF pilot peer support groups and national guidelines be developed. This was a great day! We now had to figure out how!

I began by working with a well-known Ugandan NGO, AIDS Information Center (AIC), that conducted voluntary HIV counseling and testing. I worked closely with one of their staff members who was a HIV positive mother. She became my mentor and key partner in piloting peer support groups. With her and a select team from AIC, we went into a rural health clinic to assess the interest and willingness of the HIV positive women to participate in support groups. The women were interviewed individually in private areas within the health center. During these interviews, the team members discovered how lonely and isolated the women felt. The team came together and decided to ask the women if they wanted to meet other women in the same situation that day. They all said, "Yes!" It was amazing to watch as the women met each other. I was in tears. It was clear that the support groups were critical to form.

A key question was how to roll out peer support groups nationally. It was decided that support groups could be organized at the health centers and they could meet privately in the afternoons after clinic hours. A focal person and 1 or 2 assistant(s) were selected from the existing health facility staff and trained to organize and facilitate peer support groups and to provide education on HIV/AIDS, prenatal care, postpartum care and family planning. They would meet every two weeks up to eighteen months postpartum. A standardized agenda and training materials were developed. Before or after the meetings, individual contraceptive counseling was offered to all the women. A register was developed in order to track the health care including FP of the woman.

At first the main purpose of the groups was to support HIV positive prenatal/postnatal mothers by providing an opportunity to meet and support each other psychologically, socially and to link them with HIV/AIDS prevention, care and treatment services. Later, we realized these groups needed to expand to their families and children so the groups were called PMTCT Family Support groups (FSGs). During the pilot phase, free antiretroviral drugs were becoming available so the objectives of the group incorporated the use of antiretroviral therapy (ART).

The objectives were for members to help each other to:

1. Disclose to each other, partners and children, in order to build a personal support system.
2. Accept and understand their HIV status and learn how to live positively.
3. Make informed family planning and reproductive health decisions.
4. Encourage partners and family members to get tested for HIV.
5. Learn how and when to access ARV therapy.
6. Prepare for adherence to ARVs.
7. Link and access HIV prevention, care and treatment, and support services including community services.

We decided to pilot them at four sites: two large government hospitals and two health centers which were already being supported by EGPAF.

I was able to join many support groups and listen to their life stories/testimonies. I learned a lot about the complexities of their lives. One support group member shared that when she came to the prenatal clinic and tested HIV positive, she was encouraged to disclose to her husband and to encourage him to be tested. He tested positive but to complicate matters, he had 2 other wives who now needed to be tested. The member also shared that she and her baby were treated and her baby tested HIV negative. She said, "praise to God." Another support group member shared that when she was pregnant and learned she was HIV positive, she encouraged her husband to be tested and he tested negative. They were a discordant couple. She is now on treatment and they use condoms to prevent transmitting HIV from her to her husband.

Pilot studies showed that FSGs are an essential component of the PMTCT program. Preliminary data showed that FSGs increase the uptake of Nevirapine, hospital deliveries, and family planning. Qualitative data through testimonies and observations revealed that peer support brought hope, encouraged families to stay together, improved relationships between health providers and clients, and dispelled myths and rumors regarding family planning methods. As the FSG members came to accept their diagnosis they learned more about antiretroviral therapy. The groups were linked to local resources for food supplementation, food security programs and income generating activities, family planning, and ART services.

In September 2006, just before I left Uganda, National Guidelines for Implementation of Family Support Groups in Prevention of Mother to Child Transmission of HIV were approved, printed, and disseminated! These guidelines gave a step-by-step approach on how to create and implement support groups. The guidelines were designed for the FSG focal persons responsible for organizing the groups both at the district and health facility level. The physician in charge of the PMTCT program conducted the official dissemination of the guidelines to a large audience of PMTCT stakeholders. She officially thanked EGPAF and myself for our contribution.

As a result of the video conference and the pilot FSGs, EGAF assisted the MOH to expand the FSGs. At the time that I left Uganda, seventy-five Family Support groups were established serving 4,000 women. Later I was invited by EGPAF in Mozambique and in Rwanda to introduce peer support groups in their countries.

One of my biggest compliments came from the EGPAF Scientific advisor who at first was not convinced of the importance of support groups, but before I left Uganda, she wrote, "I want to thank you for your extraordinary work. You have done a fabulous job for the foundation, teaching all of us a great deal!

Other tools to Strengthen Family Planning within the PMTCT Program

I gave technical assistance to a group of consultants who developed a five-day training handbook to update health providers in family planning knowledge and skills in order to strengthen FP within the PMTC program.

I organized and facilitated a committee which developed "A Guide to Counseling on Family Planning Methods," which is for health care providers to use in the clinic. This guide is in a flip chart format which includes a separate page for each birth control method and describes the mechanism of action, advantages, side effects and disadvantages, list of conditions of women who can and cannot use the method, and instructions for use and signs of problems that need medical attention.

I helped to develop the "My HIV Counseling Guide for PMTCT Clients", a laminated checklist for those providers counseling clients being tested for HIV. This includes one page on pre-test counseling, one on post-test counseling for HIV negative clients, and another page on post-test counseling for those HIV positive. Family Planning was included on each page.

Cross-Pollinating Ideas

Having worked in different countries, I could share their work with other countries. Before I left Uganda, I showed the head of the Reproductive Health Unit the Women's Health Care Passport used in Malawi. This passport was a simple handheld medical record where all of a woman's health information could be recorded. She was to keep it and bring it to every visit since health records were difficult to keep, maintain, and retrieve. The head of the Reproductive Health of the Ministry wanted to adapt it to Uganda and a local NGO agreed to pilot it throughout a two-year period. I was now a cross-pollinator of ideas!

Self-Entertainment

I love to be outdoors and found ways to be outside and feel personally safe.

Golfing

There were many golf courses in the country, probably because the weather was near perfect year-round. I loved golfing because it allowed me to walk in a beautiful green lush environment without hassle of street vendors. Since there were no electric carts, golfers walked and hired a caddy to carry their golf bag. My caddies were generally very good golfers who would give me advise. I tipped them well.

There were two 18-hole golf clubs where I played, one in Kampala and one in Entebbe less than an hour away. I tried to play golf every weekend and got my handicap of 34, which meant I was not very good, but that I was not a beginner. I competed in a women's international golf competition in Kampala, where I was the only white woman, and came in second to last. I was not the best golfer, but thoroughly enjoyed the game!

Once I played with a friend on the course in Fort Portal in northern Uganda. The fairways were narrow and the rough was really rough!   We found it funny we had to hire a person to run ahead of us with the flag to put in the hole on the green. This was to prevent the flags from being stolen!

Drifa was one of my golf buddies and good friend. She was Icelandic and worked for Icelandic aid (ICEADA). I told her I wanted to play golf in Nairobi for my birthday. We booked a flight and flew to Nairobi and played at the Nyeri Golf Club, a well-known golf club. In order to play on that course, you had to have a handicap and they accepted mine! It was a stunningly beautiful course.

All the golf courses I played on had beautiful trees with exotic birds such as different types of hornbills. On the course in Entebbe, I golfed near a zoo and could see white rhinos grazing in the field. There were always baby monkeys and their mothers to watch for they loved the fairways and greens of the golf courses. On the golf course in Kampala, there were lots of Marabou storks. On one occasion, I was using a yellow golf ball and a Marabou stork thought it was food and ate it. I was scared for the bird; my friend was worried how to score!

National Parks, Gorilla, and Chimpanzee treks

I went on a gorilla trek! I went with Drifa and some friends visiting from Washington State. We walked with a guide and bushwhacked into the forest for about a mile and found the gorillas. We sat very quietly for an hour watching babies with their mothers and we even saw a very large silverback, an older adult male gorilla. This was a real highlight for me.

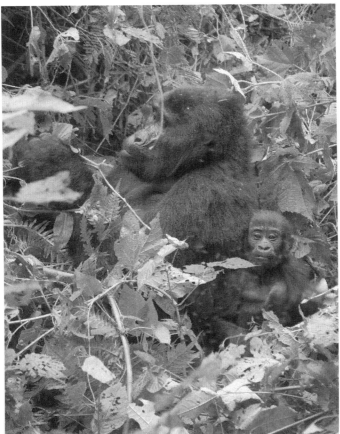

I tracked mountain gorillas in Bwindi, National Park in Uganda.
Photo by Carolyn Skye

I went on many chimpanzee treks. The Kibale Forest is home to around 1,500 chimpanzees. I went with my niece who had come to stay with me in Uganda for three months. We saw a group of large males from one troop surrounding and threatening a single male from another troop who was lying on the ground. I was very uncomfortable being there and not feeling very safe.

On another chimp trek, I went with friends to Queen Elizabeth National Park where I had to walk across a log over a rushing large river to see baby chimps. I really wanted to see them, but I was petrified of crossing over the river but there was no other way. I was very impressed with our guide. The guide took my backpack over to the other side and then came and got me. He said, "put your hands on my shoulders, walk behind me, and don't look down." I did as he said and it was well worth it. My friends and I just lay under some trees and watched the baby chimps play above us!

I also liked walking safaris. You had to go with a guide who usually carried a gun. My niece and I took a walking safari looking for a hyena den. The den was empty, but we spotted them on a nearby hill. We just sat and watched them with our binoculars. A perfect way to watch hyenas!

There were many national parks in Uganda. When my cousin and her son came to visit, we hired a guide and visited some of them. We loved sitting on the roof of the Jeep for better viewing. At the end of the trip, we were to tip the guide. I was still new to the country and didn't know how much to give him. We obviously tipped him well, because the guide called me one day and thanked me for helping him to buy his own shop in the park!

Leaving Uganda

When my contract in Uganda was up, I decided to leave international work and relocate back to the United States. While still living in Uganda, during a three-week summer vacation, I bought a house in Bristol, Vermont. Bristol was a small town of 3,800 people and reminded me of nearby Middlebury, where I grew up. I felt it was time to build a community of friends and to do all the outdoor activities while I was physically able to do them.

I lived in Bristol for almost three years. I moved into my new home with all my household effects. I met wonderful new friends and reconnected with friends I had grown up with in Middlebury. I worked as a quality assurance nurse at Home Health and Hospice. I renewed my love of kayaking and hiking and celebrated my sixtieth birthday party with a live band. I had no intention of returning to international work.

Tanzania
September 2009–December 2015

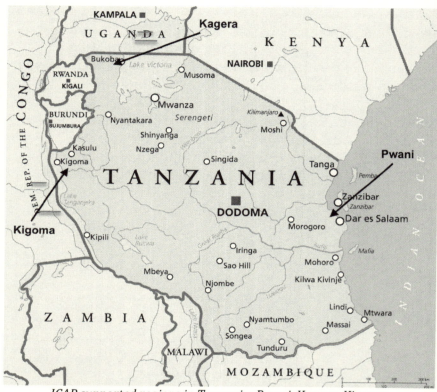

ICAP supported regions in Tanzania: Pwani, Kagera, Kigoma.

My Next Position Found Me

While I was working at Home Health and Hospice in Vermont, I got a surprise call from Amy Cunningham, who had been working for USAID in Uganda and was responsible for overseeing my work. She explained she had left USAID and was now the country director for ICAP, an international organization based out of Columbia University's School of Public Health. She called to ask me if I would come to Tanzania and provide technical assistance to her staff on how to set up Prevention of Mother to Child Transmission (PMTCT) Family Support Groups (FSGs). She wanted to replicate the Uganda program in Tanzania!

I had never heard of ICAP, which originally was an acronym for International Center for AIDS Care and Treatment Programs. I read that it was started in 2003 to address the AIDS epidemic and ICAP had offices in many other countries. The organization is now just called ICAP.

Settling In

I arrived in Dar es Salaam with Sasha and Snoops. I booked myself into the lovely Alexander's Hotel, where I stayed until I found a house to rent.

The hotel sent Stan, an English-speaking Tanzanian taxi driver, to pick me up at the airport with my luggage and pets. Little did I know that Stan would become my trusted taxi driver and friend for the rest of my years in Tanzania. I highly recommend when living in developing countries to find a driver you trust and try to avoid riding with unknown taxi drivers.

Stan helped me in many ways. For the first few months, he drove me to and from work and around Dar es Salaam until I felt confident to drive myself. He helped me to find and buy a reconditioned Toyota Corona. I always hired him to take me to and from the airport because this was the route where thieves knew you had luggage and when you were at a stop light, they would open your doors and steal your luggage. Stan was always cautious and made sure the doors were locked and windows shut. He made my trips enjoyable by introducing me to popular African music and teaching me about the culture. At one point, I learned he was a chief of one of the tribes from Mwanza!

Tanzania has many different tribes, each with its own traditions and customs. The Maasai was the name of a well-known tribe in northern Tanzania. The men came to Dar es Salaam to earn money. I was told Maasai were the best guards, reliable and trustworthy. While staying at Alexander's, I was very impressed with the kindness of one Maasai guard. Every morning and evening, I would walk Snoops on the dirt roads around the hotel. I was always worried about loose dogs attacking us. One day, as I was looking for a stick for protection, this young Maasai came up to me and offered me his walking stick. I felt so privileged and grateful! I later learned this was highly unusual for a Maasai to give anyone their stick. I treasured it for years. Sadly, I left it behind during one Christmas holiday while staying at a safari lodge in the southern highlands in Tanzania. The staff there tried to find it, but it was not to be found.

After a few weeks, I identified a two-story house to rent. It had two bedrooms and two baths on the first floor. On the second floor it had an open space for the living and dining room with big windows and a separate kitchen with a door that opened onto a large outdoor deck. Below the deck was a separate apartment for a housekeeper. I also had a small guesthouse with a thatched roof.

The house had all the security measures I was now accustomed to, except I did not have a separate metal gate to the bedroom to lock at night. I tried to install one, but the structure of the house didn't allow for it. This always bothered me due to my experience in Malawi.

I had a big yard with a beautiful flame tree which produced long lasting orange-red blooms with yellow, burgundy, or white markings. It is said to be the world's most colorful tree. I also had lots of aloe vera plants. Since I had a big yard, I built a chicken coop and had a dozen chickens so I could have fresh eggs.

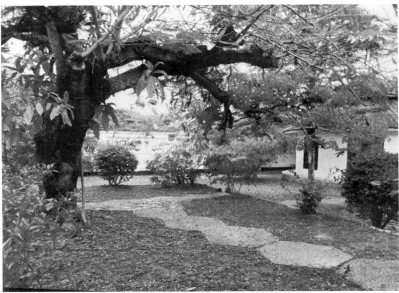

The flame tree in my yard near the thatched-roofed guesthouse.

I hired a full-time housekeeper who also was a cook and lived in the apartment below the deck. I paid her well and she enjoyed the security, yard, and free utilities. I loved and trusted her until I came home one day and found my computer missing! When she saw me panicking, she went to get her son who brought me my computer. He confessed he was using it when I was not home. I was totally surprised to learn that her son was living in a tiny storage room in the back of the house, that she allowed him in the house, and that he was borrowing my computer! Even though I got my computer back, I had to let my housekeeper go. It hurts when you bond with the people you employ and then your trust is broken.

I hired another housekeeper, who was not a cook, who remained with me until I left Dar es Salaam. I no longer needed someone to cook because I discovered Thai, Ethiopian, Indian, and Korean restaurants which all served excellent and inexpensive food! I also found well- stocked grocery stores and fruit and vegetable stands nearby so I could easily shop, prepare, and cook food for myself.

After I was living in the house, I discovered two major problems: the water source and the generator. The landlord had my water pumped up from his storage tank which was half a mile down the road. One day I had no water, so I walked down the road and was shocked to see my pipe exposed and taped closed. Someone was using my water. I called my landlord and he dug a deeper trench for the pipe and put a meter on my line. I was then charged for only the water I used and he could better track the water that was being siphoned off.

My generator was an antique and was always breaking down. This was a huge problem because the electricity would go off for hours and sometimes days. This meant no pumped water for flushing toilets, bathing, and cleaning, no cooking on the electric stove, and no air conditioning needed to sleep during hot nights. I tried to get the landlord to buy a new generator, but because they were expensive, he just kept trying to fix it.

I found very colorful and venomous caterpillars living outside my front door. One day, I put my bag down by the front door to unlock it. Unknowingly a caterpillar got on my bag which I then carried into the house. The next day, I picked up my bag to go to work and it stung me! I screamed; it was so painful that I was afraid I would die. My housekeeper came running, killed the caterpillar, put it in a bag, and off we went to an international clinic run by two Dutch physicians. We gave the bagged caterpillar to the nurses, who seemed to be more fascinated by this caterpillar than my leg, however, I was quickly reassured that I wouldn't die. They gave me some pain pills and applied lidocaine cream on my leg. Throughout the next couple of days, my leg became swollen, red, and tender. I went back to the clinic; my leg had become infected and I was immediately put on antibiotics. From that day on, I was always watching out for those caterpillars at my front door!

Work Experience

Tanzania had twenty-one regions which the government assigned to different NGOs to support their HIV/AIDS care and treatment services. ICAP was assigned by the government to support three regions: Pwani, Kigoma, and Kagera regions (see map). Dar es Salaam is located in Pwani where the main ICAP office is located and where I lived. Kagera and Kigoma were remote regions which I reached by flying in small airplanes. Kagera and Kigoma had their own separate ICAP offices, staff, and vehicles.

I always traveled with ICAP staff who were fluent in English and Kiswahili. Even though I hired a Peace Corps Tanzania language instructor and took private tutoring in Kiswahili, I did not become proficient in the language and always needed an interpreter at work. There were other tribal languages spoken, so sometimes even the ICAP staff had to find someone local to interpret.

Establishing Prevention of Mother to Child Transmission (PMTCT) Family Support Groups (FSGs)

The first few years at ICAP were devoted to establishing PMTCT Family Support Groups. I worked with two dedicated Tanzanian physicians to develop a PMTCT Family Support Group Implementation Guide with a training manual for nurses. The guide described a step-by-step process of how to set up support groups and the training manual standardized the information given in the groups. There was also a register developed that recorded each member's health care. Similar to Ugandan support groups, they were held at government health centers, after clinic hours for privacy, and were led by nurses selected as focal persons.

Once the PMTCT Family Support Group guide and a training manual were finalized, the next step was to train ICAP staff to establish the support groups. Since ICAP had field offices in three regions, it was decided to hire and train a family support group field officer for each office. The ICAP field officer's role was to assist the health centers to establish their own support groups. Before I left ICAP, there were a total of sixty-two family support groups. Since ICAP only supported three of the twenty-one regions, ICAP trained other local and international NGOs so they could establish family support groups in their assigned regions.

There were many meetings with the Ministry of Health to advocate for a national program as we had in Uganda but without success. One of the main issues was the government felt they would have to pay extra money to the nurses who took on the role of family support group focal persons even though ICAP did not pay extra allowances.

The ICAP office in Rwanda was also interested in establishing national PMTCT family support groups. I was invited to spend three weeks in Rwanda providing technical assistance. I really enjoyed my visit working with ICAP staff. I have to mention that Barack Obama won the U.S. presidential election while I was working there! I was the only American in the ICAP office and wanted to find a way to celebrate. I went to a bakery early in the morning, bought a cake, and had Obama's name written on it. With the cake in hand, I danced into the different ICAP offices. Everyone was so happy and so excited that the United States had elected a Black president! We then all gathered to share the cake and celebrate.

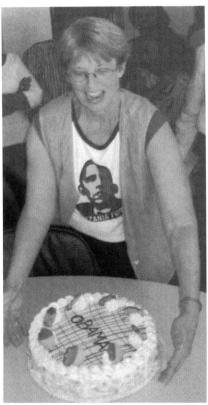

Celebrating President Barack Obama's election at ICAP in Rwanda.

Establishing a National Cervical Cancer Screening (CCS) Program

Background

Studies show that HIV positive women are at increased risk of precancerous cervical lesions and have a more rapid progression to cervical cancer. Data shows that Tanzania has one of the highest cervical cancer incidence rates in the world and the highest in East Africa. Cervical cancer is a major public health issue due to a limited access to cervical cancer screening. Pap smears, a common screening test, is not a feasible way to screen for cervical cancer due to lack of trained personnel, equipped labs, and a recall system for women who need follow-up care.

Cervical Cancer Screening Using VIA

Amy Cunningham, the ICAP/Tanzania country director, heard that Grounds for Health, an NGO from Vermont, was in Kigoma, teaching a new cervical cancer screening and treatment technique. The screening is called VIA or Visual inspection with Acetic Acid (Vinegar), a screening method that has been shown to be comparable to a pap smear. This procedure involves wiping the cervix with 5 percent white vinegar which turns precancer areas of the cervix white. The health care worker can see these white areas and treat them with cryotherapy, which is freezing the white areas with carbon dioxide (CO_2) using a cryogun. The advantages of using this method of screening is that the supplies for VIA and the CO_2 for cryotherapy are available locally and women can be screened and treated in the same visit.

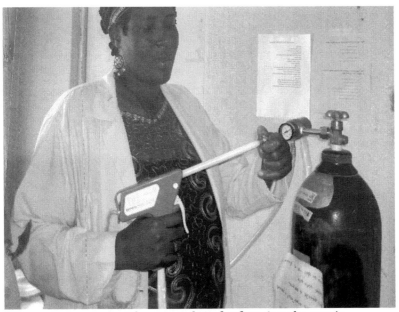

A cryogun with a special tip for freezing the cervix.
The cryogun is attached to a tank filled with CO2.

Grounds for Health was in Kigoma because it received money from free trade coffee companies to prevent cervical cancer among women coffee growers. Coffee was a major crop in this region. They were training staff in the government health centers that were located near the coffee plantations. These were the same health centers which ICAP was supporting HIV/AIDS care and treatment services. Amy thought that ICAP might want to expand this service to the other health centers in the region. She asked me to attend the training. I had heard of this technique and as a nurse practitioner in women's health care, I was excited to learn.

Grounds for Health hired a physician who had worked for the National Cancer Institute in Dar es Salaam, and now with JHPIEGO, to conduct this training. I attended the training and was trained alongside Dr. Safina Yuma, the national program officer responsible for the cervical cancer prevention and control program of the Reproductive and Child Health (RCH) section of the Ministry of Health. As a result of this training, I became very good friends with both doctors. Later they asked me to join the Ministry of Health's technical working group to develop national cervical cancer screening prevention policies, five-year strategic plans, service delivery guidelines, a monitoring information system, and information, education and communication materials.

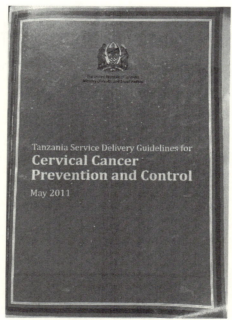

Tanzania Service Delivery Guidelines for Cervical Cancer Prevention and Control.

With ICAP support, Amy gave me the responsibility to expand cervical cancer screening in hospitals and health centers in Kigoma and then later in Kagera and Pwani. In order to do this,

I helped the ICAP staff to select and hire a cervical cancer screening officer for each of the three regional offices. I identified and ordered all the necessary equipment for the health centers. One of the biggest challenges was transporting heavy large tanks of carbon dioxide gas from a company in Dar es Salaam to the health centers in the regions. Each health center needed two tanks, so when one tank was empty there was one ready to use. Every center also needed a cryogun (see photo) to attach to the tank. The cryoguns were expensive and had to be imported from the United States.

I then worked with the Ministry of Health and JHPIEGO and expanded cervical cancer screening services through training of national trainers, supervisors, and providers in forty-three health facilities in the three ICAP-supported regions. There were other NGOs who were establishing cervical cancer screening in their government-assigned regions. When there was more than 200 clinics in the country offering cervical cancer screening, the government decided to incorporate the cervical cancer screening data into the National Health Information System (HMIS). This was a great indicator of national commitment and a sustainable program.

Experiences Traveling in the Three ICAP-Supported Regions

Kigoma

I loved traveling to the ICAP field offices in Kigoma and Kagera. Kigoma is situated along Lake Tanganyika, the second deepest and longest freshwater lake in the world. Our cervical cancer screening trainings were conducted in the Jane Goodall Institute which was on the shore of the lake. One day, while training at the Institute, one of the trainers and I were asked if we would like to meet Jane Goodall. I excitedly said, "Yes!" We were escorted to her home and talked with her for about twenty minutes! I only remember her telling us that she was a vegetarian. I thanked her for the use of her Institute for our trainings. We were fortunate to meet her because she only comes a couple times a year. On another visit, I was able to travel up Lake Tanganyika to visit her chimpanzees! There I met the people in charge of overseeing her research and the care of the chimps. That was a thrill!

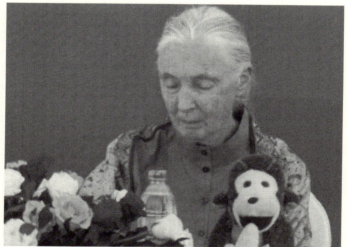

Jane Goodall giving a talk in Dar es Salaam which I attended.

In Kigoma, the ICAP staff took me to visit the Livingston Museum and monument in Ujiji. This was a place where Sir Henry Stanley rescued Dr. David Livingston, both famous nineteenth century African explorers. Dr. Livingston had been missing in Africa for four years while searching for the source of the Nile River. After a long and difficult journey, Stanley finally met and formally greeted Dr. Livingston with the famous saying, "Dr. Livingston, I presume."

154

It took almost a full day to travel to and from Kigoma. First, I would take a large commercial flight to Mwanza, a city along Lake Victoria, and then fly in a small plane to Kigoma. I had an interesting experience one day when traveling back. I was sitting with Dr. Yuma in the small airport lounge in Kigoma wondering why our plane was delayed. We learned that the airplane battery was not charged. We watched as the pilot carried the battery back and forth from the plane through the airport lounge trying to charge it. When we finally boarded, the pilot still could not start the plane. At this time, another small plane landed. We were surprised when our pilot jumped out, ran to the newly-landed plane, took its battery, put it in our plane, and started it. We were even more surprised when he returned the battery to the other plane! We took off for Mwanza with a dead battery! He was a real "bush" pilot! Thankfully, we landed safely in Mwanza.

Kagera

Kagera region was another beautiful region where I worked and traveled frequently. However, to get there, I had to fly in a small plane over Lake Victoria which could be a very bumpy ride in bad weather, but if you caught the early morning flight, it was usually a smooth ride with gorgeous sunrises! In the small planes, there was normally just one pilot and you could request to sit in the co-pilot seat. I always tried to get this seat so I could see Lake Victoria and the remote islands with the many fishing villages.

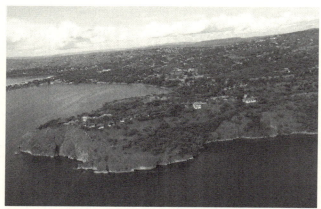

A view of Kagera from my plane. Kagera was situated on Lake Victoria.

I always stayed at this one lovely guesthouse. It had the most gorgeous garden of flowers and fruits which attracted many colorful birds. After a day of work, I would sit on the deck with a beer and my binoculars and just enjoy the view and wildlife. In the mornings, I would get up early to watch the sunrise over the lake. I felt I was in heaven!

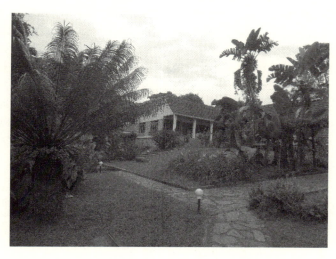

The guesthouse, my home away from home in Kagera.

It was while I was at the Kagera guesthouse that I got a phone call and learned that my friend, Ross Langdon, and his pregnant wife, Elif Yavuz, were shot and killed in the Westgate mall in Nairobi. I knew Ross well because he stayed at my home many times before he was married. He was a young architect from Tasmania and came to Africa to design buildings using local materials and which were eco-friendly. He designed the renovations of the Dar es Salaam Yacht Club which enhanced the look and function of the club. Elif was from the Netherlands, a Harvard graduate, who had just received her Ph.D. and was doing research on vaccines for the Clinton Foundation in Tanzania. They had an apartment in Dar es Salaam and had gone to Nairobi for the delivery of their first baby. They were eating in a restaurant in the mall when it was attacked by militants who killed sixty-seven people including them! After I received the phone call regarding Ross and Elif, I immediately turned on the TV and heard them talk about this tragedy and they played a video of Ross giving a "Tedx Talk" on his unique designs. It was so hard to believe they were both shot and killed.

One of the hardest times for me was when Elif's mother came to Tanzania and stayed with me while she packed out their belongings from their apartment. It was so hard to see the apartment which was fully prepared for the baby, including a crib Ross had made. I helped her by packing up all the baby clothes and distributing them to the nearby orphanages and hospitals.

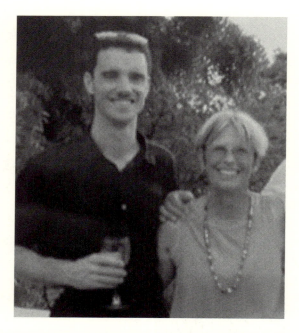

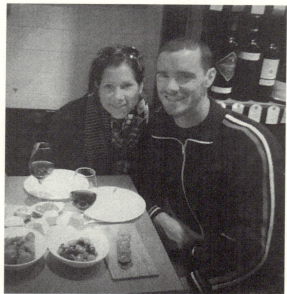

Ross and I on my deck.
Ross and his wife Elif were killed at the Westgate Mall in Nairobi.

Pwani

The third ICAP supported region was Pwani. Since the main ICAP office was in Pwani, I did not have to fly! ICAP had four-wheel drive vehicles with drivers available to take us to the health centers and hospitals. We would go for several days traveling on rough dirt roads. I always brought food to share with everyone in the car since there was not a lot of places to eat along the way. Everyone seemed to enjoy my tuna fish wraps, hard-boiled eggs, and granola bars, which I could buy in Dar Es Salaam.

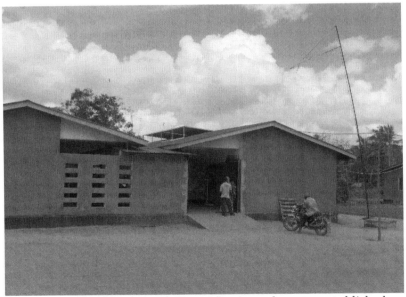

A remote health center in Pwani Region, where we established PMTCT support groups and cervical cancer screening.

I was able to enjoy the long, white sandy beaches of the coast of Pwani with friends on weekends and holidays. These beaches were not far from Dar es Salaam. We would rent cottages and spend time swimming, walking the beaches, and identifying shells. You could also find special protective netting on the beach which was placed by local villagers to protect the green turtles' eggs. A NGO called "Sea Sense" taught the villagers the importance of and how to protect the turtles and their eggs. The villagers knew when they would hatch and with Sea Sense assistance, would organize a time when the public could watch. I went several times to see the eggs hatch; what a thrill to see the baby turtles dash to the sea!

Self-Entertaining

I immediately joined the Dar es Salaam Yacht Club (DYC), located on a beautiful bay on the Indian Ocean. It has a white sandy shallow beach that is great for swimming. There are lots of different boats for fishing, sailing, and scuba diving moored there. The club house has good outdoor restaurants and a bar with outdoor seating overlooking the bay. I loved spending time there, exploring the intertidal life, kayaking, snorkeling, sailing and watching spectacular sunsets from the quarter deck. Sadly, even though the yacht club was a short walk from my house, I usually drove the five minutes because it was too dangerous to walk. There were cars or three-wheel vehicles which would drive by and grab your purse, computer, or backpack.

I love sailing and have sailed most of my life. When I joined the club, I really wanted to sail, but was not in a position to buy a boat. One day I met Mark, who was looking for a female skipper for his boat in order to compete in the annual Mermaid Cup. With fear and trepidation, I volunteered to skipper. With support from the crew, I surprised myself and everyone else when we won that race! After that, I was one of Mark's permanent crew and raced every Saturday. One time we raced to Zanzibar and spent the night. I was nervous sailing so far from shore, but I loved seeing the dolphins at our bow leading the way. I think they liked our music! We lost this race, but our crew went on to win many races!

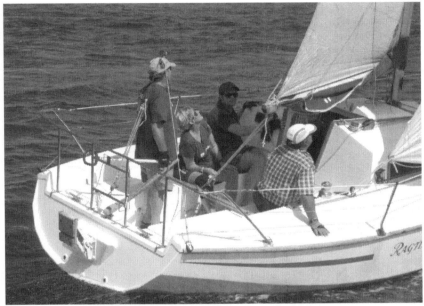

Linda crewing with Mark at the helm.

Snorkeling was amazing. The commodore of DYC, Brian, and his wife, Charlotte, were good friends and almost every Sunday they invited me to join them and others to sail on their catamaran. We sailed to remote islands where snorkeling was spectacular. I discovered a whole other world underwater! I loved the fish in the beautiful and varied coral reefs. However, we witnessed the results of dynamite fishing which was not controlled at this time. Dynamite fishing destroyed some of the coral reefs and many fish were killed unnecessarily.

Kayaking was another favorite activity. I bought a sit-upon two-person fiberglass kayak. I loved getting up early in the morning to kayak with friends before work! I later was elected the chair of the kayak committee and was instrumental in creating a formal kayak section of the yacht club. Our committee organized all kinds of activities, green-up day on remote islands, kayaking to restaurants, kayak Christmas caroling, and moonlight kayaking. These activities and more are still going on!

When I was elected as the entertainment member of the yacht club committee, I stepped down from chair of the kayak section. I was now responsible for organizing all the social events, which included classes on how to tie basic knots, identifying types of shells, and discussions on such topics as the poaching of elephants and protecting the turtles. Since I was on the DYC committee for more than two years, I am proud to say this qualified me to become a lifetime member!

Exploring Tanzania

I was fortunate to meet other single women who loved to explore Tanzania. We went to Mikumi National Park many times since it was close to Dar es Salaam. It was very sad and disturbing to see the elephant population dwindle there due to poaching. In Mkomazi National Park, it was a thrill to see the African orange bellied parrots in baobab trees! One of the women was an expert birdwatcher, so this was usually the focus of our trips. We went to Kitulo Plateau National Park, which is at 8,500 feet, to look for and find wild orchids. Botanists call this the Serengeti of Flowers.

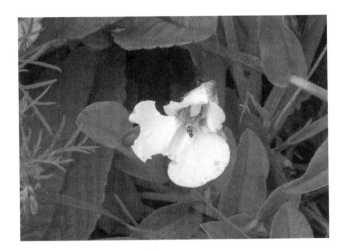

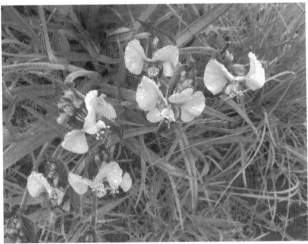

Wild orchids in Kitulo Plateau National Park.

Going to the Foxes Farm Highland Lodge for Christmas became a tradition among my expat friends. It was a two-day drive from Dar Es Salaam to this 2,000-acre working farm high up in the African Rift Valley escarpment. It was surrounded by large tea estates.

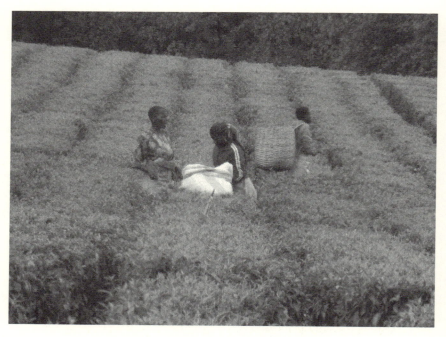

Tea estates near Foxes Farm in Mufindi.

We gathered at the highland lodge to eat our meals, and in the evenings we sat in front of a huge fireplace playing games and putting together jigsaw puzzles. We spent the night in smaller cabins on the hillside. What I loved to do was watch an elderly man command his border collies to herd the sheep! We did a lot of hiking, bird watching, and tried some fly fishing. On Christmas Eve we sang carols and on Christmas morning we had stockings and presents in one of the cabins which had a fireplace. On Christmas Day, all the guests were invited to an orphanage, supported by the farm, to see them perform the Christmas pageant, and in the evening we had a wonderful dinner at the lodge. It was all very special.

On one Christmas, a best friend from Vermont came to visit. We traveled to Foxes Farm where we had Christmas and then added a trip to Ruaha National Park which became my favorite of the parks. It was not crowded with people and the landscape was particularly beautiful with rivers, rocks, trees, and wide-open spaces where there were herds of elephants. We had a cabin with a deck right over a river where we could sit and watch hippos, elephants and other wildlife.   One of my favorite memories was on a safari drive, when we saw this stunning male lion overlooking his pride. It reminded me of Aslan the Lion in the "Narnia" series.

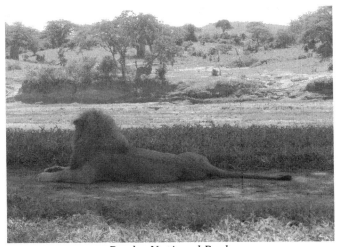

Ruaha National Park.

Leaving My Position With ICAP/Tanzania

I loved Tanzania and the people with whom I worked. I really didn't want to leave, but I had helped to start programs that were now well established and expanding. The ICAP FSG field officers were expanding the number and size of the PMTCT Family Support groups and the ICAP cervical cancer screening field officers were expanding the number of health centers offering cervical cancer screening.

Both Snoops and Sasha died while I was in Tanzania; Snoops died at age 14 and was buried in my yard with her favorite toys. Sasha died at age 22. He had stopped eating and the vet said he would not survive a flight back to the U.S. It was a very sad day when I had put him to sleep. The vet's secretary cremated Sasha in her backyard and had a wooden box made for his ashes. The vet wrote a certificate so I could bring the ashes home with me. I spread them at my favorite hiking area near my home in Vermont.

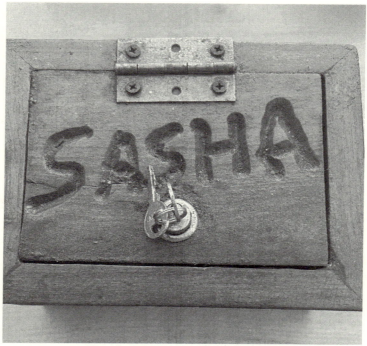

Handmade box for Sasha's ashes.

Tanzania
March to December 2016

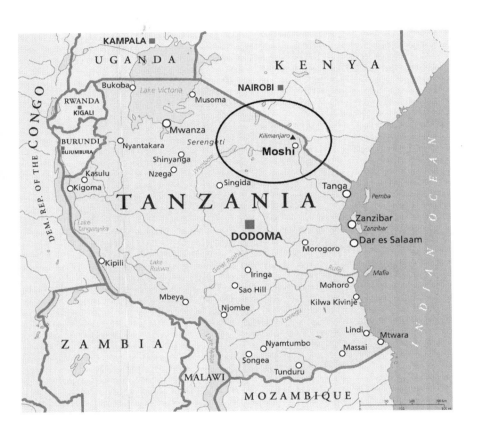

Finding My Position

Near the end of my contract with ICAP, Dr. Morales, the current Country Director of ICAP/Tanzania, introduced me to Dr. Karen Yeates, who worked for Queen's University in Kingston, Ontario, Canada. She was designing a project to scale up the use of the smartphone to improve/enhance VIA (Visual

Inspection with Acetic Acid). This project was called SEVIA (Smartphone Enhanced VIA).

When I was introduced to Dr. Yeates, I was eager to hear about SEVIA. I shared with her the work done by the Ministry of Health (MOH), JHPIEGO, and ICAP to roll out VIA to three regions. I gave her all the contacts I had that could assist her in scaling up SEVIA. I explained I worked closely with Dr. Yuma, the national program officer for cervical cancer screening, and that she was an amazingly hard worker, dedicated to the program, and key to rolling out any interventions regarding cervical cancer screening.

It took me by surprise when Dr. Yeates called me and wanted to hire me to be the SEVIA program coordinator. I, of course, was thrilled! Since my ICAP contract was ending, it was perfect timing! I would be working with a small Tanzanian NGO funded by a Canadian NGO affiliated with Queen's University. Since the local NGO had its office in Moshi, I would have to move there. Moshi was a small city in northern Tanzania in the foothills of Mount Kilimanjaro and I looked forward to exploring this part of Tanzania.

Settling In

Since I knew I was returning for a short-term assignment, I shipped most of my household effects back to Vermont, stored what I needed for Moshi, and sold the rest. I loaned my car to a friend until I returned. During the time I was away, I had friends who were kind enough to watch Shona, a Jack Russell, whom I had adopted after Snoops died.

The move was relatively easy. During the first few months in Moshi, I shared a townhouse with a colleague until I found my own home, which was a lovely old, one-story, colonial style house outside of town. It had a wonderful wraparound porch from which I had a spectacular view of Kilimanjaro! I loved it!

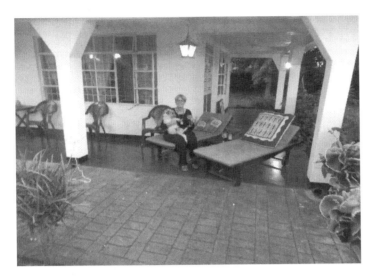

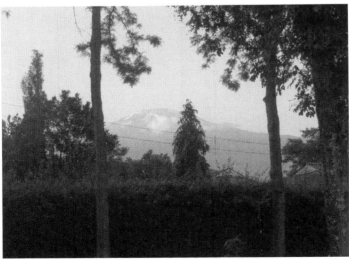

Home in Moshi with Shona. My view of Mount Kilimanjaro.

I hired a gardener to live in a small apartment next to the garage. However, I was not very lucky with my first gardener. One day I returned home after a long field trip to find my car was gone! I was stunned! My guard told me the gardener had taken the car; he thought I had given him permission to drive it. Eventually the gardener drove back and was surprised to find me home! I fired him immediately. I later learned that he had been driving around with friends and family whenever I was traveling. He did not even have a license! I was glad my car was not damaged and no one was hurt.

The next gardener I hired had a wife who was pregnant. They were extremely poor and were so appreciative of having a place to live. I made sure she had good prenatal care and I drove her and her husband to the hospital when she went into labor. Dr. Yeates was very kind and gave them the necessary baby clothes they needed. When the baby came home, I learned they had named the baby Linda. I had named three African babies through the years: Pat, Molly, and Rita, and now one was named after me!

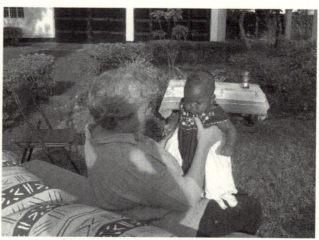

My sister-in-law with baby Linda.

I hired a wonderful English-speaking housecleaner who lived in a nearby village. She helped me communicate with the gardeners who could not speak English. We became good friends. I felt honored to be invited to her home for a meal and to meet her family.

When I arrived in Moshi, I did not know anyone except Dr. Yeates, who was very busy with many different research projects. I felt very lonely and did not have a lot of time to make friends outside of work. Fortunately, one evening when I was walking my dog, a young woman asked, "Are you Linda Andrews?" This took me by surprise. She told me she had heard I was coming through my friends at the Dar es Salaam Yacht Club and she wanted me to meet her mother-in-law, Carolyn, who was my age. I was excited to meet her.

When we met, Carolyn and I immediately became good friends. She was born of British parents, grew up in Tanzania, fluent in Kiswahili, married and raised her son and grandchildren in Tanzania. She had lived in many parts of Tanzania, but now owned a home near her son, daughter-in-law, and grandkids in Moshi. My home was located near hers, so most evenings after work, I would stop to have an evening cocktail in her backyard. Sometimes we would go to dinner at the local golf club or to her favorite Indian restaurant. I loved hearing her stories of living in Tanzania.

I discovered that living outside Moshi there was a lot to see and hear in terms of wildlife. There were lots of different birds including very noisy hornbills. It was fun to watch the bush babies jumping in the trees in the evening. I saw my first African pygmy hedgehog one evening when I was being driven home by Dr. Yeates. It was in the middle of the road, so she stopped and asked me if I would move it off the road. I was quite hesitant, it looked like it had many quills. She reassured me it was harmless. I gingerly picked it up with my hands and moved it to the side of the road. It curled up in a ball and was easy to move. I read that the quills, called spikes, are actually rigid hollow hairs, they do not have barbs like a porcupine. I later became aware that there were many hedgehogs in my yard! Most upsetting to me was that Shona liked to chase and catch them. When I would hear their loud squeal, I would run and separate the hedgehog and Shona. I found it was safest to just pick Shona up by the tail. This way, Shona immediately let go of the hedgehog and could not bite me. Thank heaven she was a Jack Russell, light and small and easy to pick up. I never found a dead hedgehog, so I think they learned to stay clear of Shona.

Work Experience

My new position as the SEVIA program coordinator was to scale up the use of the smartphone when screening for cervical cancer. SEVIA involved taking a picture of the cervix with the smartphone after the provider swabbed the cervix with 5 percent vinegar. This picture of the cervix was sent to an image reviewer who would immediately assess it and send back any recommendation for treatment. In this way, cervical cancer screening with VIA was enhanced/improved using a smartphone.

The purpose of the project was to learn lessons on how SEVIA could be expanded to a national level. A pilot study had been conducted in a nearby hospital by a team of researchers from Queen's University with Tanzanian collaborators. The study showed the rapid improvement and maintenance of skills for cervical cancer screening among health providers and led to significant improvement in the accuracy of their diagnosis. It also demonstrated that this technology could be used to mentor health service providers from remote sites.

This project's target was to screen 10,000 women for cervical cancer using the SEVIA method. I had to do this in nine months! This was a very stressful time for me trying to design the project to meet this target. In addition, we couldn't even start until we had approval by the Tanzania's National Institute for Medical Research.

To compound my stress, I had very little staff support to help me manage the finances. To relieve some of the stress, I asked Dr. Yeates and, thankfully, got her approval to hire a part-time accountant. I was so fortunate to find Juma, who was just the right person. He would sit for hours with me day and night developing budgets, reconciling budgets, and making sure we had all the proper receipts. He got special permission from his security firm, with whom he worked part time, to travel with me to five regions and to take care of paying the trainers, per diems for trainees, supplies, cars, drivers, etc. He was honest and trustworthy. Most importantly, he was always calm which kept me calm. As I got to know him, I learned he had been president and a top student in his accounting class!

I was very excited when Dr Yeates asked Dr. Yuma to be the principal investigator for the scale-up of the use of smartphones and she agreed! She helped us to select five regions for the scale-up; three of these regions were the ICAP supported regions where I already knew the cervical cancer screening supervisors, trainers, and providers. The other two regions were ones where I had never worked; Kilimanjaro Region, where I was now living, and Arusha, a neighboring region. Since Dr. Safina Yuma was the national program officer for cervical cancer, she was the right person to introduce Dr.

173

Yeates and I to the government regional officers and get the necessary approvals for this project.

In preparation for SEVIA, Dr. Yeates hired the SEVIA trainers who had conducted the pilot study. Two of these trainers were nationally respected obstetrician/gynecologists who would oversee the program, review the smartphone pictures/images, and train providers.

With Dr. Yuma's input, each region selected a SEVIA supervisor. The supervisors then selected the health facilities and the health providers to be trained. I worked closely with the supervisors to organize the SEVIA trainings. We collected baseline data six months prior to screening with the smartphone and then collected data after six months using the smartphone.

Our local NGO office had a very small space where I had a table and chair. We did not have a conference room, so I met the trainers at the local coffee shop. It was a great place to meet because you could buy freshly ground Kilimanjaro coffee and eat good food.

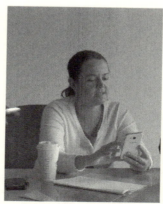

Dr. Yeates, from Queen's University, demonstrating the smartphone used in the SEVIA scale-up project.

With the SEVIA trainers that had conducted the pilot, we developed a training curriculum and tested a smartphone app, trained nine national SEVIA trainers, fourteen image reviewers, five regional SEVIA supervisors, and seventy providers in thirty-five sites in five regions in the use of smartphone. We screened 9,285 women. At the end of my contract, the government had the ability to scale-up nationally.

In addition to working within the government health facilities, we trained providers for Marie Stopes, a British supported NGO in Tanzania. Our team also traveled to Ghana to train Marie Stopes providers in SEVIA.

Near the end of my contract, Dr. Yuma visited me in Moshi and told me that the new Minister of Health had put funds in the national budget for cervical cancer screening! This meant they did not have to rely on outside funding. This was great news! Cervical cancer screening using VIA and cryotherapy was now a national program!

In regard to the use of a smartphone, the government would have to rely on outside funds to purchase the smartphones, but they did recognize that the use of the smartphone would enhance the quality of screening and be a great tool for training new providers and support for providers in the rural areas.

Follow-Up

I returned almost two years later after I had recuperated from being treated for cancer to visit friends and colleagues in Dar and Moshi. It was so wonderful to see everyone. I was honored when Dr. Safina came to my guesthouse in Dar es Salaam and spent the whole afternoon updating me on the cervical cancer screening. The program was going well.

I flew to Moshi, stayed with my friend, Carolyn, and had lunch with two of the SEVIA trainers. I was really pleased to learn that the providers we had trained in SEVIA were still using the smartphone. The image reviewers, who had been paid under our project, were mandated by the government to read the images! After lunch, the trainers took me to a market and bought a beautiful African cloth as a present for me. I was touched! I also went to see Juma, the accountant I had hired, and he was happy and doing well.

Self-Entertainment

I was so fortunate to have met Carolyn. She had become manager of Lake Chala Safari Lodge and Campsite. She invited me many times to stay with her at the lake. When there were no quests, I had the privilege to stay in the deluxe tents. The tents were built on a hill with great views of the bush and so many birds to watch from the deck.

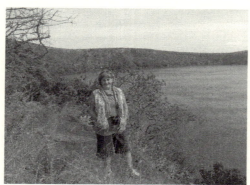

My friend, Carolyn, manager of Lake Chala Safari Lodge.

When Carolyn moved into the manager's house, I had my own room. Since she spoke fluent Kiswahili, she was very comfortable talking with the staff and local villagers. She loved living in the "bush." We drove around in her old Land Rover looking for watering holes and any signs of elephants in the area. We found honey hives in wooden barrels hanging from the trees. One day when we were walking, we saw fresh leopard tracks in the mud of the riverbank and we immediately walked back to the car. I swam and kayaked in Lake Chala, a clear deep lake which was a former volcanic crater. It was a very steep climb down and back, so I did not go often. There were many yellow baboons that would troop through the camp. I respected them and kept my distance. One evening, we saw a baboon carrying her dead baby. Later I learned that baboon mothers have been seen cradling and grooming their dead babies for up to ten days and male baboons have been seen protecting the corpses of their young from others.

My first year in Tanzania, my brother Jim, his wife Kris, some of their friends, and I explored Ngorongoro crater, Serengeti National Park, and Zanzibar. Knowing this would be my last year in Tanzania, I invited Jim and Kris to visit me in Moshi to visit a wildlife refuge, Lake Chala, and to tour three more national parks: Mkomazi, Arusha, and Tarangire.

We had some memorable moments. On the way to the wildlife refuge, we saw a dead civet on the road. I had never seen a civet before, they are rare to see because they are solitary and nocturnal. We stopped and moved it off the road so we could study this beautiful animal. We later read that their diets consist of insects and fruit, including coffee cherries. Most interesting is that an exotic and very expensive coffee is made from wild civet feces!

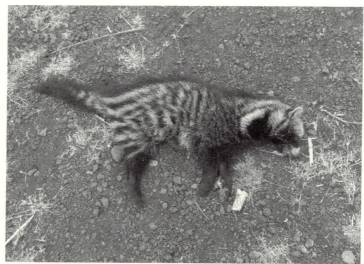
A wild civet, rarely seen, that had been hit by a vehicle.

After the wildlife center, we went to Lake Chala. We all stayed in the deluxe safari tents on the hill. I had not seen a scorpion in these tents when I stayed in them, but sure enough there was one in Jim and Kris's tent! We then traveled from Lake Chala to Mkomazi National Park and then on to Arusha and Tarangire National Parks.

We visited Lake Natron in Arusha which was a lake full of pink flamingoes! It is reported to be the home of 2.5 million Lesser Flamingoes, one of the largest pink flamingoes' breeding grounds in the world! With Jim and Kris, we were always focused on identifying birds; one day we were so focused on birds that we almost missed a pride of lions that was right on the side of the road! Our driver was so excited, he got on the radio and told all the other tour drivers. We continued birdwatching!

Leaving Moshi

My contract ended in December 2016. It was a good time to leave Tanzania when cervical cancer screening had become a funded national program and a system was in place for a national roll out of SEVIA.

I was sad to leave my friends and colleagues. I was also sad to leave Shona due to new plane restrictions. I found a great home for her on a farm with a family that wanted a companion for their Jack Russell. Before I left Tanzania, I flew to Dar es Salaam to say goodbye to friends and to crew in a final sailing race with my former captain. Stan drove me to the airport and I said my final goodbye.

United States, Vermont
December 2016

I retired from my role in international health in December 2016 and feel blessed that I was able to fulfill my lifetime dream of an international health career. Every day I learned something new and different. I feel privileged to have worked with such wonderful people from many different cultures. Though I never lived and worked in India as my grandparents did, I had a fulfilling and exciting career.

I looked forward to moving back to Vermont to reconnect with friends and family. However, it was hard to leave the work that had given me purpose and satisfaction for so many years. I grieved the loss of my international career and wondered what I could do now to contribute to my community here.

Fortuitously, as I was recovering from my cancer treatment, I heard there was an opening to elect a town chair of the Bristol Democratic Committee. I decided to run for the position and invited all my friends to vote for me; I won. This was the beginning of a new journey.

Through educational forums organized by the Bristol Democratic Committee, I learned a lot about current health care issues. As a result, I became involved in addressing the opioid crisis and the unaffordability and accessibility of health care for many Vermonters. I made a new business card, identified myself as a public health care advocate, and got to work.

When addressing these health issues, I realized the skills I learned internationally could now be used locally: identify health care needs, learn from the experts and those affected, and build a team to plan and work together to implement change. Above all, I found it critical to build trusting and respectful relationships with all interested parties. Going forward, I am committed to continuing work on health care issues and to collaborate with other people to improve the quality of life for Vermonters.

I am grateful to my parents and grandparents who supported and enabled me to have the educational opportunities and experiences I needed for this international career. I am thankful for my health and the excellent health care I received when diagnosed with cancer. I am most thankful for my family and friends who supported me through hard times so that I can continue the work I love to do in Vermont.

Acknowledgements

I am grateful for the amazing, hardworking, dedicated, and kind colleagues I worked together with in my career in international health.

Thanks to my brothers, Joel and Jim Andrews and their families who, in so many ways supported my work and my life choices.

Thanks to Dr. Shira Louria, PsyD. Clinical Psychologist at the UVM Medical Center, who encouraged me to write this memoir when I was going through chemotherapy.

Thanks to Lorrie Byrom, who sat with me during my cancer treatments, helped write my first draft of stories, suggested the title, wrote the forward, and provided many edits along the way.

Thanks to the Bristol community in Vermont for their contributions:

- Susanne Peck, artist and friend, who contributed the painting for the cover of this book.

- Christina Koliander, who edited my book and made many useful suggestions to improve clarity.

- Karen Swanson, who designed the cover, formatted the memoirs for publication, and helped me through the publishing process.

- Diana Bigelow and Jim Stapleton, who urged me to complete my memoirs and edited key sections, and Helen Young who gave me insightful comments.

Made in the USA
Middletown, DE
08 April 2023